RENAL DIET COOKBOOK FOR BEGINNERS

Comprehensive Guide With 3600 Days of Tasty, Low Sodium, Potassium, and Phosphorus Recipes for Kidney Health.

3 Weeks Meal Plan & Shopping List Included

By

Wilda Buckley

© Copyright 2023 – Wilda Buckley - All rights reserved.

This document provides exact and reliable information regarding the topic and issues covered. The publication is sold with the idea that the publisher is not required to render accounting, officially permitted or otherwise qualified services. If advice is necessary, legal, or professional, a practiced individual in the profession should be ordered.

- From a Declaration of Principles which was accepted and approved equally by a Committee of the American Bar Association and a Committee of Publishers and Associations.

In no way is it legal to reproduce, duplicate, or transmit any part of this document in either electronic means or printed format. Recording this publication is strictly prohibited, and any storage of this document is not allowed unless written permission from the publisher. All rights reserved.

The information provided herein is stated to be truthful and consistent, in that any liability, in terms of inattention or otherwise, by any usage or abuse of any policies, processes, or directions contained within is the solitary and utter responsibility of the recipient reader. Under no circumstances will any legal responsibility or blame be held against the publisher for any reparation, damages, or monetary loss due to the information herein, either directly or indirectly.

Respective authors own all copyrights not held by the publisher.

The information herein is solely offered for informational purposes and is universal. The presentation of the information is without a contract or any guarantee assurance. The trademarks used are without any consent, and the trademark publication is without permission or backing by the trademark owner. All trademarks and brands within this book are for clarifying purposes only and are owned by the owners, not affiliated with this document.

Table of Contents

INTRODUCTION 6
   How Does Kidney Work 6
   Causes 6
   What Renal Failure Can Cause? 6
   Sodium, Potassium and Phosphorous Roles in Our Body ... 6

RENAL DIET 8
   How Does It Work? 8
   Benefits 8
   Foods to Eat and To Avoid 9

21 – DAY MEAL PLAN 11

BREAKFAST 13
1. Breakfast Salad from Grains and Fruits 13
2. French toast with Applesauce 13
3. Bagels Made Healthy 13
4. Cornbread with Southern Twist 14
5. Grandma's Pancake Special 14
6. Very Berry Smoothie 14
7. Pasta with Indian Lentils 14
8. Apple Pumpkin Muffins 15
9. Spiced French Toast 15
10. Breakfast Tacos 15
11. Mexican Scrambled Eggs in Tortilla 16
12. American Blueberry Pancakes 16
13. Raspberry Peach Breakfast Smoothie 16
14. Fast Microwave Egg Scramble 16
15. Mango Lassi Smoothie 17
16. Breakfast Maple Sausage 17
17. Summer Veggie Omelet 17
18. Raspberry Overnight Porridge 17
19. Cheesy Scrambled Eggs with Fresh Herbs 18
20. Turkey and Spinach Scramble on Melba Toast ... 18
21. Vegetable Omelet 18
22. Mexican Style Burritos 18
23. Sweet Pancakes 19
24. Breakfast Smoothie 19
25. Buckwheat and Grapefruit Porridge 19
26. Egg and Veggie Muffins 19
27. Cherry Berry Bulgur Bowl 20
28. Baked Curried Apple Oatmeal Cups 20
29. Mozzarella Cheese Omelette 20
30. Sun-Dried Tomato Frittata 21
31. Italian Breakfast Frittata 21
32. Sausage Cheese Bake Omelette 21
33. Greek Egg Scrambled 21
34. Feta Mint Omelette 22
35. Sausage Casserole 22
36. Peanut Butter Bread Pudding Cups 22

SOUPS AND STEWS 23
37. Chicken Wild Rice Soup 23
38. Chicken Noodle Soup 23
39. Cucumber Soup 23
40. Squash and Turmeric Soup 23
41. Leek, Potato and Carrot Soup 24
42. Roasted Red Pepper Soup 24
43. Yucatan Soup 24
44. Zesty Taco Soup 25
45. Southwestern Posole 25
46. Spring Vegetable Soup 25
47. Seafood Corn Chowder 26
48. Beef Sage Soup 26
49. Cabbage Borscht 26
50. Ground Beef Soup 27
51. Shrimp and Crab Gumbo 27
52. Tangy Turkey Soup 28
53. Spaghetti Squash & Yellow Bell-Pepper Soup ... 28
54. Red Pepper & Brie Soup 28
55. Turkey & Lemon-Grass Soup 29
56. Paprika Pork Soup 29
57. Mediterranean Vegetable Soup 29
58. Tofu Soup 30
59. Onion Soup 30
60. Steakhouse Soup 30
61. Chinese-style Beef Stew 31
62. Stuffed Bell Pepper Soup 31
63. Salmon Chowder 31
64. Beef Stew Pasta 32
65. Italian Chicken Stew 32
66. Turkey Pasta Stew 32
67. One-Pot Chicken Pie Stew 33

FISH AND SEAFOOD 34
68. Curried Fish Cakes 34
69. Baked Sole with Caramelized Onion 34
70. Thai Tuna Wraps 34
71. Grilled Fish and Vegetable Packets 35
72. White Fish Soup 35
73. Lemon Butter Salmon 35
74. Crab Cake 36
75. Baked Fish in Cream Sauce 36
76. Shrimp & Broccoli 36

#		Page	#		Page
77.	Shrimp in Garlic Sauce	36	123.	Mixes of Snack	52
78.	Fish Taco	37	124.	Cranberry Dip with Fresh Fruit	52
79.	Baked Trout	37	125.	Cucumbers with Sour Cream	52
80.	Fish with Mushrooms	37	126.	Sweet Savory Meatballs	53
81.	Salmon with Spicy Honey	38	127.	Spicy Corn Bread	53
82.	Salmon with Maple Glaze	38	128.	Sweet and Spicy Tortilla Chips	53
83.	Steamed Spicy Tilapia Fillet	38	129.	Addictive Pretzels	54
84.	Dijon Mustard and Lime Marinated Shrimp	38	130.	Shrimp Spread with Crackers	54
85.	Baked Cod Crusted with Herbs	39	131.	Buffalo Chicken Dip	54
86.	Dill Relish on White Sea Bass	39	132.	Chicken Pepper Bacon Wraps	54
87.	Tilapia with Lemon Garlic Sauce	39	133.	Garlic Oyster Crackers	55
88.	Spinach with Tuscan White Beans and Shrimps	40	134.	Lime Cilantro Rice	55
89.	Bagel with Salmon and Egg	40	135.	Spanish Rice	55
90.	Salmon Stuffed Pasta	41	136.	Parmesan Quinoa with Peas	56
91.	Herbed Vegetable Trout	41	137.	Mushroom Orzo	56
92.	Citrus Glazed Salmon	41	138.	Carrot and Pineapple Slaw	56
93.	Broiled Salmon Fillets	42	139.	Sesame Cucumber Salad	56
94.	Broiled Shrimp	42	140.	Creamy Jalapeno Corn	57
95.	Grilled Lemony Cod	42	141.	Crispy Parmesan Cauliflower	57
96.	Spiced Honey Salmon	42	142.	Cucumber Dill Salad with Greek Yogurt Dressing	57
VEGETARIAN		**43**	143.	Zesty Green Beans with Almonds	58
97.	Tofu Stir Fry	43	144.	Dill Orzo	58
98.	Broccoli Pancake	43	145.	Quinoa Tabbouleh	58
99.	Carrot Casserole	43	146.	Papaya Mint Water	58
100.	Cauliflower Rice	44	147.	Carrot Peach Water	59
101.	Eggplant Fries	44	148.	Corn Bread	59
102.	Seasoned Green Beans	44	149.	Vegetable Rolls	59
103.	Grilled Squash	44	150.	Vegetable Fried Rice	59
105.	Thai Tofu Broth	45	151.	Tofu Stir-Fry	60
106.	Delicious Vegetarian Lasagna	45	152.	Lasagna	60
107.	Chili Tofu Noodles	45	153.	Cauliflower Patties	61
108.	Curried Cauliflower	46	154.	Turnip Chips	61
109.	Elegant Veggie Tortillas	46	**POULTRY**		**62**
110.	Simple Broccoli Stir-Fry	46	155.	Roasted Citrus Chicken	62
111.	Braised Cabbage	47	156.	Chicken with Asian Vegetables	62
112.	Salad with Strawberries and Goat Cheese	47	157.	Chicken Adobo	62
113.	Roasted Veggies Mediterranean Style	47	158.	Chicken and Veggie Soup	63
Fruity Garden Lettuce Salad		47	159.	Turkey Sausages	63
114.	Baked Dilly Pickerel	48	160.	Rosemary Chicken	63
115.	Rice Salad	48	161.	Smoky Turkey Chili	63
116.	Baked Eggplant Tray	48	162.	Avocado-Orange Grilled Chicken	64
117.	Raw Vegetables. Chopped Salad	49	163.	Herbs and Lemony Roasted Chicken	64
118.	Mediterranean Veggie Pita Sandwich	49	164.	Ground Chicken & Peas Curry	65
119.	Classic asparagus	49	165.	Chicken Meatballs Curry	65
120.	Vegetarian Pasticcio	50	166.	Ground Chicken with Basil	66
121.	Cauliflower and Asparagus Tortilla	50	167.	Chicken &Veggie Casserole	66
SNACKS AND SIDE		**52**	168.	Chicken & Cauliflower Rice Casserole	66
122.	Fluffy Mock Pancakes	52	169.	Chicken Meatloaf with Veggies	67

#	Item	Page
170.	Roasted Spatchcock Chicken	67
171.	Creamy Mushroom and Broccoli Chicken	68
172.	Chicken Curry	68
173.	Apple & Cinnamon Spiced Honey Pork Loin	68
174.	Lemon & Herb Turkey Breasts	69
175.	Beef Chimichangas	69
176.	Meat loaf	69
177.	Crockpot peachy pork chops	70
178.	Chicken avocado salad	70
179.	Chicken Mango Salsa Salad with Chipotle Lime Vinaigrette	70
180.	Chicken Salad Balsamic	71
181.	Chicken Salad with Apples, Grapes, And Walnuts	71
182.	Chicken Strawberry Spinach Salad with Ginger-Lime Dressing	71
183.	Asian Chicken Satay	72
184.	Zucchini and Turkey Burger with Jalapeno Peppers	72
185.	Gnocchi and Chicken Dumplings	72

MEAT 73

#	Item	Page
186.	Mouthwatering Beef and Chili Stew	73
187.	Beef and Three Pepper Stew	73
188.	Sticky Pulled Beef Open Sandwiches	74
189.	Herby Beef Stroganoff and Fluffy Rice	74
191.	Chunky Beef and Potato Slow Roast	75
192.	Spiced Lamb Burgers	75
193.	Pork Loins with Leeks	75
194.	Chinese Beef Wraps	76
195.	Grilled Skirt Steak	76
196.	Spicy Lamb Curry	76
197.	Lamb with Prunes	77
198.	Roast Beef	77
199.	Beef Brochettes	77
200.	Country Fried Steak	78
201.	Beef Pot Roast	78
202.	Homemade Burgers	78
203.	Slow-cooked Beef Brisket	79
204.	Pork Souvlaki	79
205.	Open-Faced Beef Stir-Up	79
206.	Grilled Steak with Cucumber Salsa	79
207.	Beef Brisket	80
208.	Apricot and Lamb Tagine	80
209.	Lamb Shoulder with Zucchini and Eggplant	81
210.	Beef Chili	81
211.	Skirt Steak Glazed with Bourbon	81

DESSERTS 83

#	Item	Page
212.	Dessert Cocktail	83
213.	Baked Egg Custard	83
214.	Gumdrop Cookies	83
215.	Pound Cake with Pineapple	83
216.	Apple Crunch Pie	84
217.	Spiced Peaches	84
218.	Pumpkin Cheesecake Bar	84
219.	Blueberry Mini Muffins	85
220.	Vanilla Custard	85
221.	Chocolate Chip Cookies	85
222.	Lemon Mousse	85
223.	Jalapeno Crisp	86
224.	Raspberry Popsicle	86
225.	Easy Fudge	86
226.	Coconut Loaf	86
227.	Chocolate Parfait	87
228.	Cauliflower Bagel	87
229.	Almond Crackers	87
230.	Cashew and Almond Butter	88
231.	Nut and Chia Mix	88
232.	Hearty Cucumber Bites	88
233.	Hearty Almond Bread	88
234.	Medjool Balls	89
235.	Blueberry Pudding	89
236.	Chia Seed Pumpkin Pudding	89
237.	Parsley Souffle	89
238.	Mug Cake Popper	90
239.	Cheesecake Bites	90
240.	Keto Mint Ginger Tea	90
241.	Keto Brownie	90
242.	Grilled Peach Sundaes	91
243.	Belgian Waffle with Fruits	91
244.	Spicy Broccoli macaroni	91
245.	Quick Quiche	91
246.	Chocolate Trifle	92
247.	Pineapple Meringues	92
248.	Baked Custard	92
249.	Strawberry Pie	92
250.	Easy Turnip Puree	93
251.	Spinach Bacon Bake	93
252.	Healthy Spinach Tomato Muffins	93

CONCLUSION 94

INTRODUCTION

How Does Kidney Work

Our kidneys are small, but they do powerful things to keep our body in balance. They are bean-shaped, about the size of a fist, and are located in the middle of the back, on the left and right sides of the spine, just below the rib cage. When everything is working properly, the kidneys do many important jobs such as:

1. Filter waste materials from the blood
2. Remove extra fluid, or water, from the body
3. Release hormones that help manage blood pressure
4. Stimulate bone marrow to make red blood cells
5. Making a vitamin D active form that promotes strong, healthy bones

Our kidneys are like a balance scale, working to keep the appropriate amounts of nutrients and minerals in the body. When the kidneys are not functioning properly, waste products and toxins will begin to accumulate in the body.

Causes

Kidney disease is most often caused by poorly controlled diabetes or high blood pressure. Physical injury and drug toxicity can also damage your kidneys. It is affecting everyone regardless of age and race, but African Americans, Hispanics, and Native Americans are studied that they have a greater risk to kidney failure. This is mostly due to a higher incidence of diabetes and high blood pressure in these populations.

Diabetes damages this process. Eventually, the kidneys cannot remove the extra waste from the blood. This ultimately leads to kidney damage or failure. This damage can happen over many years without any signs or symptoms. That's the one of the reasons why it is very important for everyone diabetes to manage their blood-sugar levels and get tested for kidney disease periodically.

Another cause of kidney disease is high blood pressure. One in three Americans with high blood pressure, also known as hypertension, is at risk for kidney disease. The second leading cause that leads to kidney disease is High blood pressure, and it increases the risk of having a heart attack/stroke. Treatment and lifestyle changes, including blood-pressure medications, following a healthy diet, and exercising can lower blood pressure.

High blood pressure means the heart has to work harder at pumping blood. As time passes, high blood pressure can harm blood vessels in your body, including the ones in your kidneys—causing them to stop filtering out waste and extra fluid from your body. The excess fluid in your blood vessels can also make your blood pressure rise, creating a vicious and detrimental cycle. As in diabetes, this damage can happen over many years without any signs or symptoms. It is very important for people with high blood pressure to control their blood pressure and get tested for kidney disease, just like people who have diabetes. High blood pressure is the cause of more than 25,000 new cases of kidney failure in the United States every year.

What Renal Failure Can Cause?

In contrast to ONN, in this disease entity kidney damage occurs gradually, primarily in the course of chronic diseases, such as:

- diabetes mellitus (diabetic nephropathy),
- hypertension (hypertensive nephropathy),
- glomerulonephritis and tubulointerstitial inflammatory processes,
- polycystic degeneration,
- systemic diseases, including sarcoidosis and amyloidosis
- less often long-term impaired blood flow or outflow of urine,
- plasma myeloma,
- HIV nephropathy
- Genetically determined syndromes, e.g., Alport syndrome.

Sodium, Potassium and Phosphorous Roles in Our Body

SODIUM

A mineral that helps regulate your body's water content and blood pressure is sodium. Healthy kidneys can remove sodium from the body as needed, but when your kidneys do not work well, sodium can build up and can cause high blood pressure, fluid-weight gain, and thirst. High blood pressure increases the chance of your kidney disease getting worse. If you are in the early stages of chronic kidney disease (stages 1 to 4), you will need to make some dietary modifications if you have high blood pressure or if you are retaining fluid. If you are experiencing stage five chronic kidney disease and require dialysis, you will need to follow a low-sodium diet and not consume more than 1,500 milligrams of sodium each day, which is equivalent to a little less than 1 teaspoon of salt. (It is important to note 1 teaspoon of salt each day is the total amount of sodium you are allowed, which includes all foods plus added salt.) Follow a sodium-restricted diet carefully to keep your blood pressure under control. Controlling your blood pressure may also prevent your risk of developing heart disease and decrease the chances of your kidney disease getting worse.

POTASSIUM

You need potassium in your body to keep your heart strong and healthy. It is also needed to keep the water balance between your cells and body fluids in check. Healthy kidneys remove excess potassium through urination. The reason why kidneys are not functioning properly is they cannot remove the potassium, so it builds up in the blood.

While some people with kidney disease need more potassium, others need less. Depending on how well your kidneys are functioning, your potassium need may vary.

All foods contain some potassium, but some foods contain large amounts of potassium. On the following pages is a table that lists low-potassium, medium-potassium, and high-potassium foods. If you have chronic kidney disease, the amount of potassium you eat is not usually restricted unless your blood potassium level is high. Please talk with your physician about having your blood potassium level checked. And if you are receiving dialysis, your potassium intake should be kept between 2,000 and 3,000 milligrams per day.

PHOSPORUS

Phosphorus is a naturally occurring mineral. Phosphates are salt compounds containing phosphorus and other minerals, and these are found in our bones. Along with calcium, phosphorus helps build strong and healthy bones. Healthy kidneys are able to remove extra phosphorus in the blood. Virtually all foods have phosphorus or phosphate additives, so it is difficult to completely eliminate it from your diet.

If you excess phosphorus in your blood, calcium is pulled from your bones, resulting in weak bones. When the kidneys are failing, phosphorus builds up in the blood and may cause problems such as severe itching, muscle aches and pain, bone disease, and hardening of the blood vessels, including those leading to the heart, as well as deposits on the skin and in the joints.

The table on the following pages lists low-phosphorus, medium-phosphorus, and high-phosphorus foods. Please talk with your physician about getting your blood phosphorus level checked.

RENAL DIET

How Does It Work?

A proper diet is necessary for controlling the amount of toxic waste in the bloodstream. When toxic waste piles up in the system along with increased fluid, chronic inflammation occurs and we will be more prone on having cardiovascular, bone, metabolic or other health issues.

Since your kidneys can't fully get rid of waste on their own, which comes from food and drinks, probably the only natural way to help our system is through this diet.

A renal diet is especially useful during the first stages of kidney dysfunction and leads to the following benefits:

- Prevents excess fluid and waste build-up
- Prevents the progression of renal dysfunction stages
- Decreases the likelihood of developing other chronic health problems e.g. heart disorders
- Has a mild antioxidant function in the body, which keeps inflammation and inflammatory responses under control.

The above-mentioned benefits are noticeable once the patient follows the diet for at least a month and then continuing it for longer periods, to avoid the stage where dialysis is needed. The strictness of the diet depends on the current stage of renal/kidney disease, if, for example, you are in the 3rd or 4th stage, you should follow a stricter diet and be attentive for the food, which is allowed or prohibited.

Benefits

Doctors and dietitians have developed a diet that helps their patients with compromised kidney function cut down the amount of waste that their body produces that their kidneys can't filter out. A renal diet is lower in sodium, phosphorus, and protein than a typical diet. Every person's body is different, which means that what works for one person will not work for another. Some people have to cut their levels of potassium and calcium as well. A renal diet must be tailored to meet the individual needs and toxin levels of the patient. Keeping a food journal may become necessary and is highly recommended. Sometimes it can be hard to keep track of all of the foods and their amounts; a journal can make keeping track a lot less intimidating. A physical notebook or even a cell phone application can be used for this.

Sodium (mg)

Sodium and table salt are two different components. Table salt is comprised of sodium and chloride. However, sodium by itself is a mineral that is naturally occurring in most of the foods that we eat. That is the reason why processed foods are not recommended for someone with kidney problems or in a renal diet due to the added salt that is put into them. Sodium is one of three major electrolytes that help control the fluids going in and out of the cells and tissue in the body. Sodium is responsible for helping control blood pressure and volume, muscle contraction and nerve functions, regulating the acid and base balance of the blood, and balancing the elimination and retention of fluid in the body.

Renal patients are required to monitor their sodium intake because when the kidney's functions become compromised, it is harder for their body to eliminate the fluids and the sodium that is in excess in the body. It has side effects that includes:

- Increased thirst
- Edema
- High blood pressure
- Shortness of breath from fluid being retained in the lungs
- Heart failure from an overworked and weak heart that has had to work harder due to the body making it work harder

Limiting sodium can be easier than you think. Since sodium content is always listed on food labels, it is important to get into the habit of checking not only sodium content but the single serving size as well. As a rule of thumb, fresh is better. Packaged foods typically have added salt, so stick with things that have no salt added to them. Start comparing the items you use. If it is a spice, steer clear of something with "salt" in the title. When you are cooking in your home, do not add extra salt to your food under any circumstance. Too much sodium can make chronic kidney disease progress much faster.

Potassium (mg)

Potassium is another of the three major electrolytes in the body. It is a naturally occurring mineral found in many foods and in our own bodies. Potassium helps keep our hearts beating regularly and our muscles working correctly. The kidneys have a duty when regulating the amount of potassium in the body. These organs, when healthy, know just how much potassium your body needs. Excess potassium is cleansed from the body through the body's urine output. When you have chronic kidney disease, this naturally occurring regulation in the body becomes compromised. Hyperkalemia, come with the following symptoms:

- Weakness in the muscles
- Irregular heartbeat
- A pulse that is slower than normal
- Heart attack/Stroke
- Death

Learning how to limit potassium, just like sodium, is an important part of your renal diet. Foods like bananas, fish, spinach, avocados, and potatoes are high in potassium and are foods to avoid. Cut down on your milk and dairy consumption to eight ounces per day. Make sure to read the labels and adhere to the single serving size of the foods you are eating.

Phosphorus (mg)

Phosphorus is a mineral that aids the bones and the muscles in the body. When food is ingested, the small intestines absorb the amount of phosphorus needed for the bones, but the kidneys are in charge of removing the extra phosphorus. When the kidneys can't expel the extra phosphorus, it builds up in the blood and pulls calcium from the bones, making them weak. High amounts of phosphorus can also cause calcium deposits to build up in the heart, lungs, eyes, and blood vessels.

Keeping phosphorus levels low, just like sodium and potassium, are important in a renal diet. Stop eating foods that are rich in phosphorus like soda, cheese, meat, milk, and seeds. It may be necessary to discuss using phosphate binders with your doctor to keep your levels under control. Make sure to avoid foods with added phosphorus. These will be labeled with "PHOS" on the label.

Protein (g)

Protein levels can be a tricky thing to keep equaled out if you have chronic kidney disease. Different stages of CKD tolerate protein levels differently and depending on which stage of CKD you are experiencing; your diet will reflect a different level of proteins allowed. Proteins are important to the body, so you can't eliminate them from your diet. You can be aware of your intake and what your body can tolerate and what it can't.

Fluid

It is important for fluid intake to be strictly monitored due to the probability of the fluid being retained in the body. When a person is on dialysis, their urine output is decreased, so extra fluid can cause unnecessary strain on the body. Fluid intake levels will be calculated by a nutritionist or doctor on a personal basis. Never drink more than what the doctor tells you is okay, and do not forget to consider solids that turn to liquid at room temperature or used in cooking.

Foods to Eat and To Avoid

When it comes to the renal diet and keeping your kidneys healthy; avoid foods that are high in:

- Potassium
- Phosphorus
- Sodium

That being said, the following food groups are strictly prohibited during a renal diet:

- Vitamin and mineral supplements
- Cheese
- Cream soup
- Dried beans/peas
- Ice cream
- Milk/coconut milk
- Nuts, low salty snack foods
- Peanut butter
- Nut butter
- Nutella

But don't be alarmed! There is still a bucket load of amazing ingredients that you can use to create awesome meals. These include:

Meat and Meat Substitutes

- Beef
- Chicken
- Fish
- Lamb
- Tuna
- Turkey
- Veal
- Pork Chops
- Tofu

Vegetables

- Beets
- Arugula
- Celery
- Chiles
- Carrots
- Asparagus
- Bean sprouts
- Chives
- Coleslaw
- Corn
- Cucumber
- Eggplants
- Endive
- Ginger root
- Green beans
- Lettuce
- Onions
- Parsley
- Radishes
- Spaghetti squash
- Turnips
- Vegetable, mixed
- Water chestnuts

Fruits

- Apricots
- Grapefruit
- Lime
- Pears
- Tangerines
- Apples
- Blackberries
- Peaches
- Pineapple
- Watermelon
- Cherries
- Figs
- Grapes
- Peach Nectar
- Raspberries
- Plums
- Apricot nectar
- Cranberries
- Fruit cocktail
- Lemon
- Pear nectar
- Strawberries

Bread and Cereals

- Corn Chex
- English muffins
- Melba toast
- Pretzels, unsalted
- Couscous
- Grits
- Noodles
- Rice/brown/white
- Kellogg's Cornflakes
- Crackers, unsalted
- Oyster crackers
- Spaghetti
- Cheerios
- Dinner rolls
- Pita Bread
- Tortillas

Fats

- Butter
- Canola oil
- Mayonnaise
- Cream cheese
- Margarine
- Miracle Whip
- Nondairy creamer
- Olive oil

Sweets

- Animal crackers
- Angel Food cake
- Candy corn
- Chewing um
- Cotton candy
- Crispy rice treats
- Graham crackers
- Gumdrops
- Gummy Bears
- Hard candy
- Hot tamales candy
- Jell-O
- Jellybeans
- Jolly Rancher
- Lemon cake
- Lifesavers
- Marshmallows
- Newtons
- Pie
- Pound cake
- Rice cakes
- Vanilla wafers

Dairy and Dairy Alternatives

- Almond milk
- Coffee-Mate
- Mocha mix
- Rice Dream
- Rich's Coffee Rich

Others

- Jelly
- Maple syrup
- Sugar, brown/white
- Honey
- Jam
- Sugar, powdered
- Corn Syrup

21 – DAY MEAL PLAN

Diets are easier when you have a definitive meal plan in your hands. This 21-day meal plan specifically for the renal diet will help you enjoy all the flavors and nutrients found in this cookbook easily.

WEEK ONE:

Day 01:
- Breakfast: Apple Onion Omelet
- Lunch: Chicken Wild Rice Soup
- Snack: Chicken Pepper Bacon Wraps
- Dinner: Braised Beef Brisket
- Dessert: Banana Pudding Dessert

Day 02:
- Breakfast: Apple Fritter Rings
- Lunch: Chicken Noodle Soup
- Snack: Snack: Chicken Pepper Bacon Wraps
- Dinner: California Pork Chops
- Dessert: Blueberry Cream Cones

Day 03:
- Breakfast: Apple Cinnamon Maple Granola
- Lunch: Cucumber Soup
- Snack: Buffalo Chicken Dip
- Dinner: Beef Chorizo
- Dessert: Cherry Dessert

Day 04:
- Breakfast: Asparagus and Cheese Crepe Rolls with Parsley
- Lunch: Squash and Turmeric Soup
- Snack: Shrimp Spread with Crackers
- Dinner: Pork Fajitas
- Dessert: Cherry Coffee Cake

Day 05:
- Breakfast: Acai Berry Smoothie Bowl
- Lunch: Wild Rice Asparagus Soup
- Snack: Garlic Oyster Crackers
- Dinner: Caribbean Turkey Curry
- Dessert: Strawberry Pie

Day 06:
- Breakfast: Baked Egg Cups
- Lunch: Nutmeg Chicken Soup
- Snack: Addictive Pretzels
- Dinner: Chicken with Rosemary-Garlic Sauce
- Dessert: Vanilla Delight

Day 07:
- Breakfast: Belgian Waffles
- Lunch: Hungarian Cherry Soup
- Snack: Sweet and Spicy Tortilla Chips
- Dinner: Chicken Fajitas
- Dessert: Chia Pudding with Berries

WEEK TWO:

Day 08:
- Breakfast: Clam Omelet
- Lunch: Italian Wedding Soup
- Snack: Spicy Corn Bread
- Dinner: Chicken with Rosemary-Garlic Sauce
- Dessert: Cranberries Snow

Day 09:
- Breakfast: Confetti Omelet
- Lunch: Old Fashioned Salmon Soup
- Snack: Sweet Savory Meatballs
- Dinner: Chicken Paprika
- Dessert: Crunchy Peppermint Cookies

Day 10:
- Breakfast: Cottage Cheese Sour Cream Pancakes
- Lunch: Oxtail Soup
- Snack: Apple Cranberry Slaw
- Dinner: Grilled Chicken Marsala
- Dessert: Apple Pie

Day 11:
- Breakfast: Apple Onion Omelet
- Lunch: Pork Fajitas
- Snack: Asian Cabbage Slaw
- Dinner: Old Fashioned Salmon Soup
- Dessert: Cherry Dessert

Day 12:
- Breakfast: Apple Fritter Rings
- Lunch: Caribbean Turkey Curry
- Snack: Autumn Orzo Salad
- Dinner: Oxtail Soup
- Dessert: Banana Pudding Dessert

Day 13:
- Breakfast: Apple Cinnamon Maple Granola

- Lunch: Chicken Fajitas
- Snack: Basil-Lime Pineapple Salad
- Dinner: Italian Wedding Soup
- Dessert: Blueberry Cream Cones

Day 14:

- Breakfast: Asparagus and Cheese Crepe Rolls with Parsley
- Lunch: Chicken with Rosemary-Garlic Sauce
- Snack: Basil-Lime Pineapple Salad
- Dinner: Hungarian Cherry Soup
- Dessert: Cherry Coffee Cake

WEEK THREE:

Day 15:

- Breakfast: Acai Berry Smoothie Bowl
- Lunch: Chicken Paprika
- Snack: Creamy Cucumber Salad
- Dinner: Nutmeg Chicken Soup
- Dessert: Blueberry Cream Cones

Day 16:

- Breakfast: Baked Egg Cups
- Lunch: Grilled Chicken Marsala
- Snack: Cucumber-Carrot Salad
- Dinner: Squash and Turmeric Soup
- Dessert: Cherry Coffee Cake

Day 17:

- Breakfast: Belgian Waffles
- Lunch: Baked Pork Chops
- Snack: Garden Vegetable Salad
- Dinner: Squash and Turmeric Soup
- Dessert: Banana Pudding Dessert

Day 18:

- Breakfast: Clam Omelet
- Lunch: Braised Beef Brisket
- Snack: Green Pepper Slaw
- Dinner: Cucumber Soup
- Dessert: Apple Pie

Day 19:

- Breakfast: Confetti Omelet
- Lunch: California Pork Chops
- Snack: Cranberry Cream Salad
- Dinner: Chicken Noodle Soup
- Dessert: Strawberry Pie

Day 20:

- Breakfast: Apple Onion Omelet
- Lunch: Baked Pork Chops
- Snack: Creamy Cucumber Salad
- Dinner: Chicken Wild Rice Soup
- Dessert: Vanilla Delight

Day 21:

- Breakfast: Cottage Cheese Sour Cream Pancakes
- Lunch: Squash and Turmeric Soup
- Snack: Cucumber-Carrot Salad
- Dinner: Baked Pork Chops
- Dessert: Apple Pie

BREAKFAST

1. Breakfast Salad from Grains and Fruits

Preparation time: 5 minutes

Cooking time: 15 minutes

Servings: 6

INGREDIENTS:

- 1 8-oz low fat vanilla yogurt
- 1 cup raisins
- 1 orange
- 1 Red delicious apple
- 1 Granny Smith apple
- ¾ cup bulgur
- ¾ cup quick cooking brown rice
- ¼ teaspoon salt
- 3 cups water

DIRECTION:

1. On high fire, place a large pot and bring water to a boil.
2. Add bulgur and rice. Lower fire to a simmer and cooks for ten minutes while covered.
3. Turn off fire, set aside for 2 minutes while covered.
4. In baking sheet, transfer and evenly spread grains to cool.
5. Meanwhile, peel oranges and cut into sections. Chop and core apples.
6. Once grains are cool, transfer to a large serving bowl along with fruits.
7. Add yogurt and mix well to coat.
8. Serve and enjoy.

NUTRITION: Calories: 187; Carbs: g; Protein: g; Fats: g; Phosphorus: mg; Potassium: mg; Sodium: 117mg

2. French toast with Applesauce

Preparation time: 5 minutes

Cooking time: 15 minutes

Servings: 6

INGREDIENTS:

- ¼ cup unsweetened applesauce
- ½ cup milk
- 1 teaspoon ground cinnamon
- 2 eggs
- 2 tablespoon white sugar
- 6 slices whole wheat bread

DIRECTIONS:

1. Mix well applesauce, sugar, cinnamon, milk and eggs in a mixing bowl.
2. Dip the bread into applesauce mixture until wet, take note that you should do this one slice at a time.
3. On medium fire, heat a nonstick skillet greased with cooking spray.
4. Add soaked bread one at a time and cook for 2-3 minutes per side or until lightly browned.
5. Serve and enjoy.

NUTRITION: Calories: 57; Carbs: 6g; Protein: 4g; Fats: 4g; Phosphorus: 69mg; Potassium: 88mg; Sodium: 43mg

3. Bagels Made Healthy

Preparation time: 5 minutes

Cooking time: 25 minutes

Servings: 8

INGREDIENTS:

- 2 teaspoon yeast
- 1 ½ tablespoon olive oil
- 1 ¼ cups bread flour
- 2 cups whole wheat flour
- 1 tablespoon vinegar
- 2 tablespoon honey
- 1 ½ cups warm water

DIRECTIONS:

1. In a bread machine, mix all ingredients, and then process on dough cycle.
2. Once done or end of cycle, create 8 pieces shaped like a flattened ball.
3. Using your thumb, you must create a hole at the center of each then create a donut shape.
4. In a greased baking sheet, place donut-shaped dough then covers and let it rise about ½ hour.
5. Prepare about 2 inches of water to boil in a large pan.
6. In a boiling water, drop one at a time the bagels and boil for 1 minute, then turn them once.
7. Remove them and return them to baking sheet and bake at 350oF (175oC) for about 20 to 25 minutes until golden brown.

NUTRITION: Calories: 221; Carbs: 42g; Protein: 7g; Fats: g; Phosphorus: 130mg; Potassium: 166mg; Sodium: 47mg

4. Cornbread with Southern Twist

Preparation time: 15 minutes
Cooking time: 60 minutes
Servings: 8

INGREDIENTS:
- 2 tablespoons shortening
- 1 ¼ cups skim milk
- ¼ cup egg substitute
- 4 tablespoons sodium free baking powder
- ½ cup flour
- 1 ½ cups cornmeal

DIRECTIONS:
1. Prepare 8 x 8-inch baking dish or a black iron skillet then add shortening.
2. Put the baking dish or skillet inside the oven on 425oF, once the shortening has melted that means the pan is hot already.
3. In a bowl, add milk and egg then mix well.
4. Take out the skillet and add the melted shortening into the batter and stir well.
5. Pour mixture into skillet after mixing all ingredients.
6. Cook the cornbread for 15-20 minutes until it is golden brown.

NUTRITION: Calories: 166; Carbs: 35g; Protein: 5g; Fats: 1g; Phosphorus: 79mg; Potassium: 122mg; Sodium: 34mg

5. Grandma's Pancake Special

Preparation time: 5 minutes

Cooking time: 15 minutes

Servings: 3

INGREDIENTS:
- 1 tablespoon oil
- 1 cup milk
- 1 egg
- 2 teaspoons sodium free baking powder
- 2 tablespoons sugar
- 1 ¼ cups flour

DIRECTIONS:
1. Mix together all the dry ingredients such as the flour, sugar and baking powder.
2. Combine oil, milk and egg in another bowl. Once done, add them all to the flour mixture.
3. Make sure that as your stir the mixture, blend them together until slightly lumpy.
4. In a hot greased griddle, pour-in at least ¼ cup of the batter to make each pancake.
5. To cook, ensure that the bottom is a bit brown, then turn and cook the other side, as well.

NUTRITION: Calories: 167; Carbs: 50g; Protein: 11g; Fats: 11g; Phosphorus: 176mg; Potassium: 215mg; Sodium: 70mg

6. Very Berry Smoothie

Preparation time: 3 minutes

Cooking time: 5 minutes

Servings: 2

INGREDIENTS:
- 2 quarts water
- 2 cups pomegranate seeds
- 1 cup blackberries
- 1 cup blueberries

DIRECTIONS:
1. Mix all ingredients in a blender.
2. Puree until smooth and creamy.
3. Transfer to a serving glass and enjoy.

NUTRITION: Calories: 464; Carbs: 111g; Protein: 8g; Fats: 4g; Phosphorus: 132mg; Potassium: 843mg; Sodium: 16mg

7. Pasta with Indian Lentils

Preparation time: 5 minutes

Cooking time: 0 minutes

Servings: 6

INGREDIENTS:
- ¼-½ cup fresh cilantro (chopped)
- 3 cups water
- 2 small dry red peppers (whole)
- 1 teaspoon turmeric
- 1 teaspoon ground cumin
- 2-3 cloves garlic (minced)
- 1 can diced tomatoes (w/juice)
- 1 large onion (chopped)
- ½ cup dry lentils (rinsed)
- ½ cup orzo or tiny pasta

DIRECTIONS:
1. Combine all ingredients in the skillet except for the cilantro then boil on medium-high heat.
2. Ensure to cover and slightly reduce heat to medium-low and simmer until pasta is tender for about 35 minutes.
3. Afterwards, take out the chili peppers then add cilantro and top it with low-fat sour cream.

NUTRITION: Calories: 175; Carbs: 40g; Protein: 3g; Fats: 2g; Phosphorus: 139mg; Potassium: 513mg; Sodium: 61mg

8. Apple Pumpkin Muffins

Preparation Time: 15 minutes

Cooking Time: 20 minutes

Servings: 12

INGREDIENTS

- 1 cup all-purpose flour
- 1 cup wheat bran
- 2 teaspoons Phosphorus Powder
- 1 cup pumpkin purée
- ¼ cup honey
- ¼ cup olive oil
- 1 egg
- 1 teaspoon vanilla extract
- ½ cup cored diced apple

DIRECTIONS

1. Preheat the oven to 400°F.
2. Line 12 muffin cups with paper liners.
3. Stir together the flour, wheat bran, and baking powder, mix this in a medium bowl.
4. In a small bowl, whisk together the pumpkin, honey, olive oil, egg, and vanilla.
5. Stir the pumpkin mixture into the flour mixture until just combined.
6. Stir in the diced apple.
7. Spoon the batter in the muffin cups.
8. Bake for about 20 minutes, or until a toothpick inserted in the center of a muffin comes out clean.

NUTRITION PER SERVING: (1 muffin): Calories: 125; Total Fat: 5g; Saturated Fat: 1g; Cholesterol: 18mg; Sodium: 8mg; Carbohydrates: 20g; Fiber: 3g; Phosphorus: 120mg; Potassium: 177mg; Protein: 2g

9. Spiced French Toast

Preparation Time: 15 minutes

Cooking Time: 12 minutes

Servings: 4

INGREDIENTS

- 4 eggs
- ½ cup Homemade Rice Milk (here, or use unsweetened store-bought) or almond milk
- ¼ cup freshly squeezed orange juice
- 1 teaspoon ground cinnamon
- ½ teaspoon ground ginger
- Pinch ground cloves
- 1 tablespoon unsalted butter, divided
- 8 slices white bread

DIRECTIONS

1. Whisk eggs, rice milk, orange juice, cinnamon, ginger, and cloves until well blended in a large bowl.
2. Melt half the butter in a large skillet. It should be in medium-high heat only.
3. Dredge four of the bread slices in the egg mixture until well soaked, and place them in the skillet.
4. Cook the toast until golden brown on both sides, turning once, about 6 minutes total.
5. Repeat with the remaining butter and bread.
6. Serve 2 pieces of hot French toast to each person.

NUTRITION PER SERVING: Calories: 236; Total fat: 11g; Saturated fat: 4g; Cholesterol: 220mg; Sodium: 84mg; Carbohydrates: 27g; Fiber: 1g; Phosphorus: 119mg; Potassium: 158mg; Protein: 11g

10. Breakfast Tacos

Preparation Time: 10 minutes

Cooking Time: 10 minutes

Servings: 4

INGREDIENTS

- 1 teaspoon olive oil
- ½ sweet onion, chopped
- ½ red bell pepper, chopped
- ½ teaspoon minced garlic
- 4 eggs, beaten
- ½ teaspoon ground cumin
- Pinch red pepper flakes
- 4 tortillas
- ¼ cup tomato salsa

DIRECTIONS

1. Heat the oil in a large skillet in a medium heat only.
2. Add the onion, bell pepper, and garlic, and sauté until softened, about 5 minutes.
3. Add the eggs, cumin, and red pepper flakes, and scramble the eggs with the vegetables until cooked through and fluffy.
4. Spoon one-fourth of the egg mixture into the center of each tortilla, and top each with 1 tablespoon of salsa.
5. Serve immediately.

NUTRITION PER SERVING: Calories: 211; Total fat: 7g; Saturated fat: 2g; Cholesterol: 211mg; Sodium: 346mg; Carbohydrates: 17g; Fiber: 1g; Phosphorus: 120mg; Potassium: 141mg; Protein: 9g

11. Mexican Scrambled Eggs in Tortilla

Preparation Time: 5 minutes

Cooking Time: 2 minutes

Servings: 2

INGREDIENTS

- 2 medium corn tortillas
- 4 egg whites
- 1 teaspoon of cumin
- 3 teaspoons of green chilies, diced
- ½ teaspoon of hot pepper sauce
- 2 tablespoons of salsa
- ½ teaspoon salt

DIRECTIONS

1. Spray some cooking spray on a medium skillet and heat for a few seconds.
2. Whisk the eggs with the green chilies, hot sauce, and comminute
3. Add the eggs into the pan, and whisk with a spatula to scramble. Add the salt.
4. Cook until fluffy and done (1-2 minutes) over low heat.
5. Open the tortillas and spread 1 tablespoon of salsa on each.
6. Distribute the egg mixture onto the tortillas and wrap gently to make a burrito.
7. Serve warm.

NUTRITION: Calories: 44.1 kcal Carbohydrate: 2.23 g Protein: 7.69 g Sodium: 854 mg Potassium: 189 mg Phosphorus: 22 mg Dietary Fiber: 0.5 g Fat: 0.39 g

12. American Blueberry Pancakes

Preparation Time: 5 minutes

Cooking Time: 10 minutes

Servings: 6

INGREDIENTS

- 1 ½ cups of all-purpose flour, sifted
- 1 cup of buttermilk
- 3 tablespoons of sugar
- 2 tablespoons of unsalted butter, melted
- 2 teaspoon of baking powder
- 2 eggs, beaten
- 1 cup of canned blueberries, rinsed

DIRECTIONS

1. Combine the baking powder, flour and sugar in a bowl.
2. Make a hole in the center and slowly add the rest of the ingredients.
3. Begin to stir gently from the sides to the center with a spatula, until you get a smooth and creamy batter.
4. With cooking spray, spray the pan and place over medium heat.
5. Take one measuring cup and fill 1/3rd of its capacity with the batter to make each pancake.
6. Use a spoon to pour the pancake batter and let cook until golden brown. Flip once to cook the other side.
7. Serve warm with optional agave syrup.

NUTRITION: Calories: 251.69 kcal Carbohydrate: 41.68 g Protein: 7.2 g Sodium: 186.68 mg Potassium: 142.87 mg Phosphorus: 255.39 mg Dietary Fiber: 1.9 g Fat: 6.47 g

13. Raspberry Peach Breakfast Smoothie

Preparation Time: 5 minutes

Cooking Time: 1 minute

Servings: 2

INGREDIENTS

- 1/3 cup of raspberries, (it can be frozen)
- 1/2 peach, skin and pit removed
- 1 tablespoon of honey
- 1 cup of coconut water

DIRECTIONS

1. Mix all ingredients together and blend it until smooth.
2. Pour and serve chilled in a tall glass or mason jar.

NUTRITION: Calories: 86.3 kcal Carbohydrate: 20.6 g Protein: 1.4 g Sodium: 3 mg Potassium: 109 mg Phosphorus: 36.08 mg Dietary Fiber: 2.6 g Fat: 0.31 g

14. Fast Microwave Egg Scramble

Preparation Time: 5 minutes

Cooking Time: 1-2 minutes

Servings: 1

INGREDIENTS

- 1 large egg
- 2 large egg whites
- 2 tablespoons of milk
- Kosher pepper, ground

DIRECTIONS

1. Spray a coffee cup with a bit of cooking spray.
2. Whisk all the ingredients together and place into the coffee cup.
3. Place the cup with the eggs into the microwave and set to cook for approx. 45 seconds. Take out and stir.

4. Cook it for another 30 seconds after returning it to the microwave.
5. Serve.

NUTRITION: Calories: 128.6 kcal Carbohydrate: 2.47 g Protein: 12.96 g Sodium: 286.36 mg Potassium: 185.28 mg Phosphorus: 122.22 mg Dietary Fiber: 0 g Fat: 5.96 g

15. Mango Lassi Smoothie

Preparation Time: 5 minutes

Cooking Time: 0 minute

Servings: 2

INGREDIENTS

- ½ cup of plain yogurt
- ½ cup of plain water
- ½ cup of sliced mango
- 1 tablespoon of sugar
- ¼ teaspoon of cardamom
- ¼ teaspoon cinnamon
- ¼ cup lime juice

DIRECTIONS

1. Pulse all the above ingredients in a blender until smooth (around 1 minute).
2. Pour into tall glasses or mason jars and serve chilled immediately.

NUTRITION: Calories: 89.02 kcal Carbohydrate: 14.31 g Protein: 2.54 g Sodium: 30 mg Potassium: 185.67 mg Phosphorus: 67.88 mg Dietary Fiber: 0.77 g Fat: 2.05 g

16. Breakfast Maple Sausage

Preparation Time: 15 minutes

Cooking Time: 8 minutes

Servings: 12

INGREDIENTS

- 1 pound of pork, minced
- ½ pound lean turkey meat, ground
- ¼ teaspoon of nutmeg
- ½ teaspoon black pepper
- ¼ all spice
- 2 tablespoon of maple syrup
- 1 tablespoon of water

DIRECTIONS

1. Combine all the ingredients in a bowl.
2. Cover and refrigerate for 3-4 hours.
3. Take the mixture and form into small flat patties with your hand (around 10-12 patties).
4. Lightly grease a medium skillet with oil and shallow fry the patties over medium to high heat, until brown (around 4-5 minutes on each side).
5. Serve hot.

NUTRITION: Calories: 53.85 kcal Carbohydrate: 2.42 g Protein: 8.5 g Sodium: 30.96 mg Potassium: 84.68 mg Phosphorus: 83.49 mg Dietary Fiber: 0.03 g Fat: 0.9 g

17. Summer Veggie Omelet

Preparation Time: 5 minutes

Cooking Time: 5 minutes

Servings: 2

INGREDIENTS

- 4 large egg whites
- ¼ cup of sweet corn, frozen
- ⅓ cup of zucchini, grated
- 2 green onions, sliced
- 1 tablespoon of cream cheese
- Kosher pepper

DIRECTIONS

1. Grease a medium pan with some cooking spray and add the onions, corn and grated zucchini.
2. Sauté for a couple of minutes until softened.
3. Beat the eggs together with the water, cream cheese, and pepper in a bowl.
4. Add the eggs into the veggie mixture in the pan, and let cook while moving the edges from inside to outside with a spatula, to allow raw egg to cook through the edges.
5. Turn the omelet with the aid of a dish (placed over the pan and flipped upside down and then back to the pan).
6. Let sit for another 1-2 minutes.
7. Fold in half and serve.

NUTRITION: Calories: 90 kcal Carbohydrate: 15.97 g Protein: 8.07 g Sodium: 227 mg Potassium: 244.24 mg Phosphorus: 45.32 mg Dietary Fiber: 0.88 g Fat: 2.44 g

18. Raspberry Overnight Porridge

Preparation Time: Overnight

Cooking Time: 0 minute

Servings: 12

INGREDIENTS

- ⅓ cup of rolled oats
- ½ cup almond milk
- 1 tablespoon of honey
- 5-6 raspberries, fresh or canned and unsweetened
- ⅓ cup of rolled oats
- ½ cup almond milk
- 1 tablespoon of honey
- 5-6 raspberries, fresh or canned and unsweetened

DIRECTIONS

1. Combine the oats, almond milk, and honey in a mason jar and place into the fridge for overnight.
2. Serve the next morning with the raspberries on top.

NUTRITION: Calories: 143.6 kcal Carbohydrate: 34.62 g Protein: 3.44 g Sodium: 77.88 mg Potassium: 153.25 mg Phosphorus: 99.3 mg Dietary Fiber: 7.56 g Fat: 3.91 g

19. Cheesy Scrambled Eggs with Fresh Herbs

Preparation Time: 15 minutes

Cooking Time: 10 minutes

Servings: 4

INGREDIENTS

- Eggs – 3
- Egg whites – 2
- Cream cheese – ½ cup
- Unsweetened rice milk – ¼ cup
- Chopped scallion – 1 Tablespoon green part only
- Chopped fresh tarragon – 1 Tablespoon
- Unsalted butter – 2 Tablespoons.
- Ground black pepper to taste

DIRECTIONS

1. In a container, mix the eggs, egg whites, cream cheese, rice milk, scallions, and tarragon until mixed and smooth.
2. Melt the butter in a skillet.
3. Pour in the egg mix and cook, stirring, for 5 minutes or until the eggs are thick and curds creamy.
4. Season with pepper and serve.

NUTRITION: Calories: 221 Fat: 19g Carb: 3g Phosphorus: 119mg Potassium: 140mg Sodium: 193mg Protein: 8g

20. Turkey and Spinach Scramble on Melba Toast

Preparation Time: 2 minutes

Cooking Time: 15 minutes

Servings: 2

INGREDIENTS

- Extra virgin olive oil – 1 teaspoon
- Raw spinach – 1 cup
- Garlic – ½ clove, minced
- Nutmeg – 1 teaspoon grated
- Cooked and diced turkey breast – 1 cup
- Melba toast – 4 slices
- Balsamic vinegar – 1 teaspoon

DIRECTIONS

1. Heat a pot over a source of heat and add oil.
2. Add turkey and heat through for 6 to 8 minutes.
3. Add spinach, garlic, and nutmeg and stir-fry for 6 minutes more.
4. Plate up the Melba toast and top with spinach and turkey scramble.
5. Drizzle with balsamic vinegar and serve.

NUTRITION: Calories: 301 Fat: 19g Carb: 12g Phosphorus: 215mg Potassium: 269mg Sodium: 360mg Protein: 19g

21. Vegetable Omelet

Preparation Time: 15 minutes

Cooking Time: 10 minutes

Servings: 3

INGREDIENTS

- Egg whites – 4
- Egg – 1
- Chopped fresh parsley – 2 Tablespoons.
- Water – 2 Tablespoons.
- Olive oil spray
- Chopped and boiled red bell pepper – ½ cup
- Chopped scallion – ¼ cup, both green and white parts
- Ground black pepper

DIRECTIONS

1. Whisk together the egg, egg whites, parsley, and water until well blended. Set aside.
2. Spray a skillet with olive oil spray and place over medium heat.
3. Sauté the peppers and scallion for 3 minutes or until softened.
4. Over the vegetables, you can now pour the egg and cook, swirling the skillet, for 2 minutes or until the edges start to set. Cook until set.
5. Season with black pepper and serve.

NUTRITION: Calories: 77 Fat: 3g Carb: 2g Phosphorus: 67mg Potassium: 194mg Sodium: 229mg Protein: 12g

22. Mexican Style Burritos

Preparation Time: 5 minutes

Cooking Time: 15 minutes

Servings: 2

INGREDIENTS

- Olive oil – 1 Tablespoon
- Corn tortillas – 2
- Red onion – ¼ cup, chopped
- Red bell peppers – ¼ cup, chopped
- Red chili – ½, deseeded and chopped

- Eggs – 2
- Juice of 1 lime
- Cilantro – 1 Tablespoon chopped

DIRECTIONS

1. Turn the broiler to medium heat and place the tortillas underneath for 1 to 2 minutes on each side or until lightly toasted.
2. Remove and keep the broiler on.
3. Sauté onion, chili and bell peppers for 5 to 6 minutes or until soft.
4. Place the eggs on top of the onions and peppers and place skillet under the broiler for 5-6 minutes or until the eggs are cooked.
5. Serve half the eggs and vegetables on top of each tortilla and sprinkle with cilantro and lime juice to serve.

NUTRITION: Calories: 202 Fat: 13g Carb: 19g Phosphorus: 184mg Potassium: 233mg Sodium: 77mg Protein: 9g

23. Sweet Pancakes

Preparation Time: 10 minutes

Cooking Time: 5 minutes

Servings: 5

INGREDIENTS

- All-purpose flour – 1 cup
- Granulated sugar – 1 Tablespoon
- Baking powder – 2 teaspoons.
- Egg whites – 2
- Almond milk - 1 cup
- Olive oil - 2 Tablespoons.
- Maple extract – 1 Tablespoon

DIRECTIONS

1. Combine the flour, sugar and baking powder in a bowl.
2. Make a well in the center and place to one side.
3. Mix the egg whites, milk, oil, and maple extract, do this in another bowl.
4. Add the egg mixture to the well and gently mix until a batter is formed.
5. Heat skillet over medium heat.
6. Cook 2 minutes on each side or until the pancake is golden only add 1/5 of the batter to the pan.
7. Repeat with the remaining batter and serve.

NUTRITION: Calories: 178 Fat Potassium: 126mg Sodium: 297mg Protein: 6g

24. Breakfast Smoothie

Preparation Time: 15 minutes

Cooking Time: 0 minute

Servings: 2

INGREDIENTS

- Frozen blueberries – 1 cup
- Pineapple chunks – ½ cup
- English cucumber – ½ cup
- Apple – ½
- Water – ½ cup

DIRECTIONS

1. Put the pineapple, blueberries, cucumber, apple, and water in a blender and blend until thick and smooth.
2. Pour into 2 glasses and serve.

NUTRITION: Calories: 87 Fat: g Carb: 22g Phosphorus: 28mg Potassium: 192mg Sodium: 3mg Protein: 0.7g

25. Buckwheat and Grapefruit Porridge

Preparation Time: 5 minutes

Cooking Time: 20 minutes

Servings: 2

INGREDIENTS

- Buckwheat – ½ cup
- Grapefruit – ¼, chopped
- Honey – 1 Tablespoon
- Almond milk – 1 ½ cups
- Water – 2 cups

DIRECTIONS

1. Boil water on the stove. Add the buckwheat and place the lid on the pan.
2. Simmer for 7 to 10 minutes, in a lowheat. Check to ensure water does not dry out.
3. Remove and set aside for 5 minutes, do this when most of the water is absorbed.
4. Drain excess water from the pan and stir in almond milk, heating through for 5 minutes.
5. Add the honey and grapefruit.
6. Serve.

NUTRITION: Calories: 231 Fat: 4g Carb: 43g Phosphorus: 165mg Potassium: 370mg Sodium: 135mg

26. Egg and Veggie Muffins

Preparation Time: 15 minutes

Cooking Time: 20 minutes

Servings: 4

INGREDIENTS

- Cooking spray
- Eggs – 4
- Unsweetened rice milk – 2 Tablespoon
- Sweet onion – ½, chopped
- Red bell pepper – ½, chopped

- Pinch red pepper flakes
- Pinch ground black pepper

DIRECTIONS

1. Preheat the oven to 350F.
2. Spray 4 muffin pans with cooking spray. Set aside.
3. Whisk together the milk, eggs, onion, red pepper, parsley, red pepper flakes, and black pepper until mixed.
4. Pour the egg mixture into prepared muffin pans.
5. Bake until the muffins are puffed and golden, about 18 to 20 minutes.
6. serve

NUTRITION: Calories: 84 Fat: 5g Carb: 3g Phosphorus: 110mg Potassium: 117mg Sodium: 75mg Protein: 7g

27. Cherry Berry Bulgur Bowl

Preparation Time: 15 minutes

Cooking Time: 15 minutes

Servings: 4

INGREDIENTS

- 1 cup medium-grind bulgur
- 2 cups water
- Pinch salt
- 1 cup halved and pitted cherries or 1 cup canned cherries, drained
- ½ cup raspberries
- ½ cup blackberries
- 1 tablespoon cherry jam
- 2 cups plain whole-milk yogurt

DIRECTIONS

1. Mix the bulgur, water, and salt in a medium saucepan. Do this in a medium heat. Bring to a boil.
2. Reduce the heat to low and simmer, partially covered, for 12 to 15 minutes or until the bulgur is almost tender. Cover, and let stand for 5 minutes to finish cooking do this after removing the pan from the heat.
3. While the bulgur is cooking, combine the raspberries and blackberries in a medium bowl. Stir the cherry jam into the fruit.
4. When the bulgur is tender, divide among four bowls. Top each bowl with ½ cup of yogurt and an equal amount of the berry mixture and serve.

NUTRITION PER SERVING: Calories: 242; Total fat: 6g; Saturated fat: 3g; Sodium: 85mg; Phosphorus: 237mg; Potassium: 438mg; Carbohydrates: 44g; Fiber: 7g; Protein: 9g; Sugar: 13g

28. Baked Curried Apple Oatmeal Cups

Preparation Time: 10 minutes

Cooking Time: 20 minutes

Servings: 6

INGREDIENTS

- 3½ cups old-fashioned oats
- 3 tablespoons brown sugar
- 2 teaspoons of your preferred curry powder
- ⅛ teaspoon salt
- 1 cup unsweetened almond milk
- 1 cup unsweetened applesauce
- 1 teaspoon vanilla
- ½ cup chopped walnuts

DIRECTIONS

1. Preheat the oven to 375°F. Then spray a 12-cup muffin tin with baking spray then set aside.
2. Combine the oats, brown sugar, curry powder, and salt, and mix in a medium bowl.
3. Mix together the milk, applesauce, and vanilla in a small bowl,
4. Stir the liquid ingredients into the dry ingredients and mix until just combined. Stir in the walnuts.
5. Using a scant ⅓ cup for each divide the mixture among the muffin cups.
6. Bake this for 18 to 20 minutes until the oatmeal is firm. Serve.

NUTRITION: For 2 Oatmeal Cups: Calories: 296; Total fat: 10g; Saturated fat: 1g; Sodium: 84mg; Phosphorus: 236mg; Potassium: 289mg; Carbohydrates: 45g; Fiber: 6g; Protein: 8g; Sugar: 11g

29. Mozzarella Cheese Omelette

Preparation Time: 10 minutes

Cooking Time: 5 minutes

Servings: 1

INGREDIENTS:

- 4 eggs, beaten
- 1/4 cup mozzarella cheese, shredded
- 4 tomato slices
- 1/4 tsp Italian seasoning
- 1/4 tsp dried oregano
- Pepper
- Salt

DIRECTIONS:

1. In a small bowl, whisk eggs with salt.
2. Spray pan with cooking spray and heat over medium heat.

3. Pour egg mixture into the pan and cook over medium heat.
4. Once eggs are set then sprinkle oregano and Italian seasoning on top.
5. Arrange tomato slices on top of the omelet and sprinkle with shredded cheese.
6. Cook omelet for 1 minute.
7. Serve and enjoy.

NUTRITION: Calories 285 Fat 19 g Carbohydrates 4 g Sugar 3 g Protein 25 g Cholesterol 655 mg

30. Sun-Dried Tomato Frittata

Preparation Time: 10 minutes

Cooking Time: 20 minutes

Servings: 8

INGREDIENTS:

- 12 eggs
- 1/2 tsp dried basil
- 1/4 cup parmesan cheese, grated
- 2 cups baby spinach, shredded
- 1/4 cup sun-dried tomatoes, sliced
- Pepper
- Salt

DIRECTIONS:

1. Preheat the oven to 425 F.
2. In a large bowl, whisk eggs with pepper and salt.
3. Add remaining ingredients and stir to combine.
4. Spray oven-safe pan with cooking spray.
5. Pour egg mixture into the pan and bake for 20 minutes.
6. Slice and serve.

NUTRITION: Calories 115 Fat 7 g Carbohydrates 1 g Sugar 1 g Protein 10 g Cholesterol 250 mg

31. Italian Breakfast Frittata

Preparation Time: 10 minutes

Cooking Time: 45 minutes

Servings: 4

INGREDIENTS:

- 2 cups egg whites
- 1/2 cup mozzarella cheese, shredded
- 1 cup cottage cheese, crumbled
- 1/4 cup fresh basil, sliced
- 1/2 cup roasted red peppers, sliced
- Pepper
- Salt

DIRECTIONS:

1. Preheat the oven to 375 F.
2. Add all ingredients into the large bowl and whisk well to combine.
3. Pour frittata mixture into the baking dish and bake for 45 minutes.
4. Slice and serve.

NUTRITION: Calories 131 Fat 2 g Carbohydrates 5 g Sugar 2 g Protein 22 g Cholesterol 6 mg

32. Sausage Cheese Bake Omelette

Preparation Time: 10 minutes

Cooking Time: 45 minutes

Servings: 8

INGREDIENTS:

- 16 eggs
- 2 cups cheddar cheese, shredded
- 1/2 cup salsa
- 1 lb ground sausage
- 1 1/2 cups coconut milk
- Pepper
- Salt

DIRECTIONS:

1. Preheat the oven to 350 F.
2. Add sausage in a pan and cook until browned. Drain excess fat.
3. In a large bowl, whisk eggs and milk. Stir in cheese, cooked sausage, and salsa.
4. Pour omelet mixture into the baking dish and bake for 45 minutes.
5. Serve and enjoy.

NUTRITION: Calories 360 Fat 24 g Carbohydrates 4 g Sugar 3 g Protein 28 g Cholesterol 400 mg

33. Greek Egg Scrambled

Preparation Time: 10 minutes

Cooking Time: 10 minutes

Servings: 2

INGREDIENTS:

- 4 eggs
- 1/2 cup grape tomatoes, sliced
- 2 tbsp green onions, sliced
- 1 bell pepper, diced
- 1 tbsp olive oil
- 1/4 tsp dried oregano
- 1/2 tbsp capers
- 3 olives, sliced
- Pepper
- Salt

DIRECTIONS:

1. Heat oil in a pan over medium heat.

2. Add green onions and bell pepper and cook until pepper is softened.
3. Add tomatoes, capers, and olives and cook for 1 minute.
4. Add eggs and stir until eggs are cooked. Season with oregano, pepper, and salt.
5. Serve and enjoy.

NUTRITION: Calories 230 Fat 17 g Carbohydrates 8 g Sugar 5 g Protein 12 g Cholesterol 325 mg

34. Feta Mint Omelette

Preparation Time: 10 minutes

Cooking Time: 5 minutes

Servings: 1

INGREDIENTS:

- 3 eggs
- 1/4 cup fresh mint, chopped
- 2 tbsp coconut milk
- 1/2 tsp olive oil
- 2 tbsp feta cheese, crumbled
- Pepper
- Salt

DIRECTIONS:

1. In a bowl, whisk eggs with feta cheese, mint, milk, pepper, and salt.
2. Heat olive oil in a pan over low heat.
3. Pour egg mixture in the pan and cook until eggs are set.
4. Flip omelet and cook for 2 minutes more.
5. Serve and enjoy.

NUTRITION: Calories 275 Fat 20 g Carbohydrates 4 g Sugar 2 g Protein 20 g Cholesterol 505 mg

35. Sausage Casserole

Preparation Time: 10 minutes

Cooking Time: 50 minutes

Servings: 8

INGREDIENTS:

- 12 eggs
- 1 lb. ground Italian sausage
- 2 1/2 tomatoes, sliced
- 3 tbsp coconut flour
- 1/4 cup coconut milk
- 2 small zucchinis, shredded
- Pepper
- Salt

DIRECTIONS:

1. Preheat the oven to 350 F.
2. Cook sausage in a pan until brown.
3. Transfer sausage to a mixing bowl.
4. Add coconut flour, milk, eggs, zucchini, pepper, and salt. Stir well.
5. Add eggs and whisk to combine.
6. Transfer bowl mixture into the casserole dish and top with tomato slices.
7. Bake for 50 minutes.
8. Serve and enjoy.

NUTRITION: Calories 305 Fat 21.8 g Carbohydrates 6.3 g Sugar 3.3 g Protein 19.6 g Cholesterol 286 mg

36. Peanut Butter Bread Pudding Cups

Preparation Time: 10 minutes

Cooking Time: 20 minutes

Servings: 6

INGREDIENTS

- Baking spray
- 5 slices whole-wheat bread, coarsely crumbled
- 2 large eggs
- ½ cup unsweetened almond milk
- ¼ cup peanut butter
- 2 tablespoons honey
- 1 teaspoon vanilla
- ½ cup chopped unsalted peanuts

DIRECTIONS

1. Preheat the oven to 375°F. And then spray a 6-cup muffin tin with baking spray and set aside.
2. Put the breadcrumbs in a medium bowl.
3. Beat the eggs, milk, peanut butter, honey, and vanilla until smooth. Pour over the breadcrumbs.
4. Stir gently until combined, then divide the mixture evenly among the muffin cups. Sprinkle with the peanuts.
5. Bake this for 18-20 minutes or until the puddings are set. Serve warm.

NUTRITION: Per Cup: Calories: 261; Total fat: 15g; Saturated fat: 3g; Sodium: 220mg; Phosphorus: 176mg; Potassium: 261mg; Carbohydrates: 24g; Fiber: 3g; Protein: 12g; Sugar: 9g

SOUPS AND STEWS

37. Chicken Wild Rice Soup

Preparation time: 10 minutes

Cooking time: 15 minutes

Servings: 6

INGREDIENTS

- 2/3 cup wild rice, uncooked
- 1 tablespoon onion, chopped finely
- 1 tablespoon fresh parsley, chopped
- 1 cup carrots, chopped
- 8-ounce chicken breast, cooked
- 2 tablespoon butter
- 1/4 cup all-purpose white flour
- 5 cups low-sodium chicken broth
- 1 tablespoon slivered almonds

DIRECTIONS

1. Start by adding rice and 2 cups broth along with ½ cup water to a cooking pot.
2. Cook the chicken until the rice is al dente and set it aside.
3. Add butter to a saucepan and melt it.
4. Stir in onion and sauté until soft then add the flour and the remaining broth.
5. Stir it and then cook for it 1 minute then add the chicken, cooked rice, and carrots.
6. Cook for 5 minutes on simmer.
7. Garnish with almonds.
8. Serve fresh.

NUTRITION: Calories 287. Protein 21 g. Carbohydrates 35 g. Fat 7 g. Cholesterol 42 mg. Sodium 182 mg. Potassium 384 mg. Phosphorus 217 mg. Calcium 45 mg. Fiber 1.6 g.

38. Chicken Noodle Soup

Preparation time: 10 minutes

Cooking time: 25 minutes

Servings: 2

INGREDIENTS

- 1 1/2 cups low-sodium vegetable broth
- 1 cup of water
- 1/4 teaspoon poultry seasoning
- 1/4 teaspoon black pepper
- 1 cup chicken strips
- 1/4 cup carrot
- 2-ounce egg noodles, uncooked

DIRECTIONS

1. Gather all the ingredients into a slow cooker and toss it
2. Cook soup on high heat for 25 minutes.
3. Serve warm.

NUTRITION: Calories 103. Protein 8 g. Carbohydrates 11 g. Fat 3 g. Cholesterol 4 mg. Sodium 355 mg. Potassium 264 mg. Phosphorus 128 mg. Calcium 46 mg. Fiber 4.0 g.

39. Cucumber Soup

Preparation time: 10 minutes

Cooking time: 0 minutes

Servings: 4

INGREDIENTS

- 2 medium cucumbers, peeled and diced
- 1/3 cup sweet white onion, diced
- 1 green onion, diced
- 1/4 cup fresh mint
- 2 tablespoon fresh dill
- 2 tablespoon lemon juice
- 2/3 cup water
- 1/2 cup half and half cream
- 1/3 cup sour cream
- 1/2 teaspoon pepper
- Fresh dill sprigs for garnish

DIRECTIONS

1. Gather all of the ingredients into a food processor and toss.
2. Puree the mixture and refrigerate for 2 hours.
3. Garnish with dill sprigs.
4. Enjoy fresh.

NUTRITION: Calories 77. Protein 2 g. Carbohydrates 6 g. Fat 5 g. Cholesterol 12 mg. Sodium 128 mg. Potassium 258 mg. Phosphorus 64 mg. Calcium 60 mg. Fiber 1.0 g.

40. Squash and Turmeric Soup

Preparation time: 10 minutes

Cooking time: 30 minutes

Servings: 4

INGREDIENTS

- 4 cups low-sodium vegetable broth
- 2 medium zucchini squash, peeled and diced
- 2 medium yellow crookneck squash, peeled and diced
- 1 small onion, diced
- 1/2 cup frozen green peas
- 2 tablespoon olive oil
- 1/2 cup plain nonfat Greek yogurt
- 2 teaspoon turmeric

DIRECTIONS

1. Warm the broth in a saucepan on medium heat.
2. Toss in onion, squash, and zucchini.
3. Let it simmer for approximately 25 minutes then add oil and green peas.
4. Cook for another 5 minutes then allow it to cool.
5. Puree the soup using a handheld blender then add Greek yogurt and turmeric.
6. Refrigerate it overnight and serve fresh.

NUTRITION: Calories 100. Protein 4 g. Carbohydrates 10 g. Fat 5 g. Cholesterol 1 mg. Sodium 279 mg. Potassium 504 mg. Phosphorus 138 mg. Calcium 60 mg. Fiber 2.8 g.

41. Leek, Potato and Carrot Soup

Preparation time: 15min

Cooking time: 25min

Servings: 4

INGREDIENTS

- 1 - leek
- ¾ - cup diced and boiled potatoes
- ¾ - cup diced and boiled carrots
- 1 - garlic clove
- 1 - tablespoon oil
- crushed pepper to taste
- 3 - cups low sodium chicken stock
- chopped parsley for garnish
- 1 - bay leaf
- ¼ - teaspoon ground cumin

DIRECTIONS

1. Trim off and take away a portion of the coarse inexperienced portions of the leek, at that factor reduce daintily and flush altogether in virus water.
2. Channel properly. Warmth the oil in an extensively based pot.
3. Include the leek and garlic, and sear over low warmth for two-3 minutes, till sensitive.
4. Include the inventory, inlet leaf, cumin, and pepper. Heat the mixture, mix constantly.
5. Include the bubbled potatoes and carrots and stew for 10-15minutes
6. Modify the flavoring, eliminate the inlet leaf and serve sprinkled generously with slashed parsley.
7. To make a pureed soup, manner the soup in a blender or nourishment processor till smooth
8. Come again to the pan. Include ½ field milk.
9. Bring to bubble and stew for 2-3minutes

NUTRITION: Calories 315g, Fat 8g, Carbs 15g, Sugars 1.2g, Protein 26g

42. Roasted Red Pepper Soup

Preparation time: 30min

Cooking time: 35min

Servings: 4

INGREDIENTS

- 4 - cups low-sodium chicken broth
- 3 - red peppers
- 2 - medium onions
- 3 - tablespoon lemon juice
- 1 - tablespoon finely minced lemon zest
- A pinch cayenne peppers
- ¼ - teaspoon cinnamon
- ½ - cup finely minced fresh cilantro

DIRECTIONS

1. In a medium stockpot, consolidate each one of the fixings except for the cilantro and warmth to the point of boiling over excessive warm temperature.
2. Diminish the warmth and stew, ordinarily secured, for around 30 minutes, till thickened.
3. Cool marginally. Utilizing a hand blender or nourishment processor, puree the soup.
4. Include the cilantro and tenderly heat.

NUTRITION: Calories 265g, Fat 8g, Carbs 5g, Sugars 0.1g, Protein 29g

43. Yucatan Soup

Preparation time: 10 minutes

Cooking time: 20 minutes

Servings: 4

INGREDIENTS

- ½ cup onion, chopped
- 8 cloves garlic, chopped
- 2 Serrano chili peppers, chopped
- 1 medium tomato, chopped
- 1 ½ cups chicken breast, cooked, shredded
- 2 six-inch corn tortillas, sliced
- Nonstick cooking spray
- 1 tablespoon olive oil
- 4 cups chicken broth
- 1 bay leaf
- ¼ cup lime juice
- ¼ cup cilantro, chopped
- 1 teaspoon black pepper

DIRECTIONS

1. Spread the corn tortillas in a baking sheet and bake them for 3 minutes at 400ºF.

2. Place a suitably-sized saucepan over medium heat and add oil to heat.
3. Toss in chili peppers, garlic, and onion, then sauté until soft.
4. Stir in broth, tomatoes, bay leaf, and chicken.
5. Let this chicken soup cook for 10 minutes on a simmer.
6. Stir in cilantro, lime juice, and black pepper.
7. Garnish with baked corn tortillas.
8. Serve.

NUTRITION: Calories: 215 Protein: 21 g Carbohydrates: 32 g Fat: 10 g Cholesterol: 32 mg Sodium: 246 mg Potassium: 355 mg Phosphorus: 176 mg Calcium: 47 mg Fiber: 1.6 g

44. Zesty Taco Soup

Preparation time: 10 minutes

Cooking time: 7 hours

Servings: 2

INGREDIENTS

- 1 ½ pounds boneless skinless chicken breast
- 15 ½ ounces canned dark red kidney beans
- 15 ½ ounces canned white corn
- 1 cup canned tomatoes, diced
- ½ cup onion
- 15 ½ ounces canned yellow hominy
- ½ cup green bell peppers
- 1 garlic clove
- 1 medium jalapeno
- 1 tablespoon package McCormick
- 2 cups chicken broth

DIRECTIONS

1. Add drained beans, hominy, corn, onion, garlic, jalapeno pepper, chicken, and green peppers to a Crockpot.
2. Cover the beans-corn mixture and cook for 1 hour on High temperature.
3. Reduce the heat to LOW and continue cooking for 6 hours.
4. Shred the slow-cooked chicken and return to the taco soup.
5. Serve warm.

NUTRITION: Calories: 191 Protein: 21 g Carbohydrates: 20 g Fat: 3 g Cholesterol: 42 mg Sodium: 421 mg Potassium: 444 mg Phosphorus: 210 mg Calcium: 28 mg Fiber: 4.3 g

45. Southwestern Posole

Preparation time: 10 minutes

Cooking time: 53 minutes

Servings: 4

INGREDIENTS

- 1 tablespoon olive oil
- 1-pound pork loin, diced
- ½ cup onion, chopped
- 1 garlic clove, chopped
- 28 ounces canned white hominy
- 4 ounces canned diced green chilis
- 4 cups chicken broth
- ¼ teaspoon black pepper

DIRECTIONS

1. Place a suitably-sized cooking pot over medium heat and add oil to heat.
2. Toss in pork pieces and sauté for 4 minutes.
3. Stir in garlic and onion, then stir for 4 minutes, or until onion is soft.
4. Add the remaining ingredients, then cover the pork soup.
5. Cook this for 45 minutes, or until the pork is tender.
6. Serve warm.

NUTRITION: Calories: 286 Protein: 25 g Carbohydrates: 15 g Fat: 13 g Cholesterol: 63 mg Sodium: 399 mg Potassium: 346 mg Phosphorus: 182 mg Calcium: 31 mg Fiber: 3.4 g

46. Spring Vegetable Soup

Preparation time: 10 minutes

Cooking time: 45 minutes

Servings: 4

INGREDIENTS

- 1 cup fresh green beans, chopped
- ¾ cup celery, chopped
- ½ cup onion, chopped
- ½ cup carrots, chopped
- ½ cup mushrooms, chopped
- ½ cup frozen corn
- 1 medium Roma tomato, chopped
- 2 tablespoons olive oil
- ½ cup frozen corn
- 4 cups vegetable broth
- 1 teaspoon dried oregano leaves
- 1 teaspoon garlic powder

DIRECTIONS

1. Place a suitably-sized cooking pot over medium heat and add olive oil to heat.

2. Toss in onion and celery, then sauté until soft.
3. Stir in the corn and rest of the ingredients and cook the soup to boil.
4. Now reduce its heat to a simmer and cook for 45 minutes.
5. Serve warm.

NUTRITION: Calories: 115 Protein: 3 g Carbohydrates: 13 g Fat: 6 g Cholesterol: 0 mg Sodium: 262 mg Potassium: 400 mg Phosphorus: 108 mg Calcium: 48 mg Fiber: 3.4 g

47. Seafood Corn Chowder

Preparation time: 10 minutes

Cooking time: 12 minutes

Servings: 4

INGREDIENTS

- 1 tablespoon butter
- 1 cup onion, chopped
- 1/3 cup celery, chopped
- ½ cup green bell pepper, chopped
- ½ cup red bell pepper, chopped
- 1 tablespoon white flour
- 14 ounces chicken broth
- 2 cups cream
- 6 ounces evaporated milk
- 10 ounces surimi imitation crab chunks
- 2 cups frozen corn kernels
- ½ teaspoon black pepper
- ½ teaspoon paprika

DIRECTIONS

1. Place a suitably-sized saucepan over medium heat and add butter to melt.
2. Toss in onion, green and red peppers, and celery, then sauté for 5 minutes.
3. Stir in flour and whisk well for 2 minutes.
4. Pour in chicken broth and stir until it boils.
5. Add evaporated milk, corn, surimi crab, paprika, black pepper, and creamer.
6. Cook for 5 minutes then serve warm.

NUTRITION: Calories: 175 Protein: 8 g Carbohydrates: 24 g Fat: 7 g Cholesterol: 13 mg Sodium: 160 mg Potassium: 285 mg Phosphorus: 181 mg Calcium: 68 mg Fiber: 1.5 g

48. Beef Sage Soup

Preparation time: 10 minutes

Cooking time: 20 minutes

Servings: 4

INGREDIENTS

- ½ pound ground beef
- ½ teaspoon ground sage
- ½ teaspoon black pepper
- ½ teaspoon dried basil
- ½ teaspoon garlic powder
- 4 slices bread, cubed
- 2 tablespoons olive oil
- 1 tablespoon herb seasoning blend
- 2 garlic cloves, minced
- 3 cups chicken broth
- 1 ½ cups water
- 4 tablespoons fresh parsley
- 2 tablespoons parmesan cheese, grated

DIRECTIONS

1. Preheat your oven to 375ºF.
2. Mix beef with sage, basil, black pepper, and garlic powder in a bowl, then set it aside.
3. Toss the bread cubes with olive oil in a baking sheet and bake them for 8 minutes.
4. Meanwhile, sauté the beef mixture in a greased cooking pot until it is browned.
5. Stir in garlic and sauté for 2 minutes, then add parsley, water, and broth.
6. Cover the beef soup and cook for 10 minutes on a simmer.
7. Garnish the soup with parmesan cheese and baked bread.
8. Serve warm.

NUTRITION: Calories: 336 Protein: 26 g Carbohydrates: 16 g Fat: 19 g Cholesterol: 250 mg Sodium: 374 mg Potassium: 392 mg Phosphorus: 268 mg Calcium: 118 mg Fiber: 0.9 g

49. Cabbage Borscht

Preparation time: 10 minutes

Cooking time: 1 hour, 30 minutes

Servings: 6

INGREDIENTS

- 2 pounds beef steaks
- 6 cups cold water
- 2 tablespoons olive oil
- ½ cup tomato sauce
- 1 medium cabbage, chopped
- 1 cup onion, diced

- 1 cup carrots, diced
- 1 cup turnips, peeled and diced
- 1 teaspoon pepper
- 6 tablespoons lemon juice
- 4 tablespoons sugar

DIRECTIONS

1. Start by placing steak in a large cooking pot and pour enough water to cover it.
2. Cover the beef pot and cook it on a simmer until it is tender, then shred it using a fork.
3. Add olive oil, onion, tomato sauce, carrots, turnips, and shredded steak to the cooking liquid in the pot.
4. Stir in black pepper, sugar, and lemon juice to season the soup.
5. Cover the cabbage soup and cook on low heat for 1 ½ hour.
6. Serve warm.

NUTRITION: Calories: 212 Protein: 19 g Carbohydrates: 10 g Fat: 10 g Cholesterol: 60 mg Sodium: 242 mg Potassium: 388 mg Phosphorus: 160 mg Calcium: 46 mg Fiber: 2.1 g

50. Ground Beef Soup

Preparation time: 10 minutes

Cooking time: 30 minutes

Servings: 4

INGREDIENTS

- 1-pound lean ground beef
- ½ cup onion, chopped
- 2 teaspoons lemon-pepper seasoning blend
- 1 cup beef broth
- 2 cups of water
- 1/3 cup white rice, uncooked
- 3 cups frozen mixed vegetables
- 1 tablespoon sour cream

DIRECTIONS

1. Spray a saucepan with cooking oil and place it over medium heat.
2. Toss in onion and ground beef, then sauté until brown.
3. Stir in broth and rest of the ingredients, then boil it.
4. Reduce heat to a simmer, then cover the soup to cook for 30 minutes.
5. Garnish with sour cream.
6. Enjoy.

NUTRITION: Calories: 223 Protein: 20 g Carbohydrates: 20 g Fat: 8 g Cholesterol: 52 mg Sodium: 170 mg Potassium: 448 mg Phosphorus: 210 mg Calcium: 43 mg Fiber: 4.3 g

51. Shrimp and Crab Gumbo

Preparation time: 10 minutes

Cooking time: 15 minutes

Servings: 4

INGREDIENTS

- 1 cup bell pepper, chopped
- 1 ½ cups onion, chopped
- 1 garlic clove, chopped
- ¼ cup celery leaves, chopped
- 1 cup green onion tops
- ¼ cup fresh parsley, chopped
- 4 tablespoons canola oil
- 6 tablespoons all-purpose white flour
- 3 cups of water
- 4 cups chicken broth
- 8 ounces shrimp, uncooked
- 6 ounces crab meat
- ¼ teaspoon black pepper
- 1 teaspoon hot sauce
- 3 cups cooked rice

DIRECTIONS

1. Prepare the roux in a suitably-sized pan by heating oil in it.
2. Stir in flour and sauté until it changes its color.
3. Pour in 1 cup water, then add onion, garlic, celery leaves, and bell pepper.
4. Cover the roux mixture and cook on low heat until the veggies turn soft.
5. Add 2 cups water and 4 cups broth, then mix again.
6. Continue cooking it for 5 minutes then add crab meat and shrimp.
7. Cook for 10 minutes then and parsley and green onion.
8. Continue cooking for 5 minutes then garnish with black pepper and hot sauce.
9. Serve warm with rice.

NUTRITION: Calories: 328 Protein: 22 g Carbohydrates: 34 g Fat: 11 g Cholesterol: 86 mg Sodium: 328 mg Potassium: 368 mg Phosphorus: 221 mg Calcium: 79 mg Fiber: 1.4 g

52. Tangy Turkey Soup

Preparation time: 10 minutes

Cooking time: 68 minutes

Servings: 4

INGREDIENTS

- 1 cup carrots, chopped
- 1 cup celery, chopped
- 1 cup green bell pepper, chopped
- 1 cup yellow onion, chopped
- ½ cup fresh tomato, chopped
- ½ cup fresh parsley, chopped
- 2 garlic cloves, chopped
- 1 cup mushrooms, sliced
- 2 cups zucchini, sliced
- 1 tablespoon olive oil
- 1-pound turkey breast, skinless, cubed
- ½ teaspoon black pepper
- ½ cup dry white wine
- 4 cups chicken broth
- 1 teaspoon dried thyme
- 1 bay leaf
- ¼ teaspoon crushed red pepper
- 3 cups white rice, cooked
- 3 tablespoons lemon juice

DIRECTIONS

1. Place a suitably-sized stockpot over medium heat and oil to heat.
2. Toss in turkey, and black pepper, then sauté for 10 minutes.
3. Stir in green bell pepper, onion, celery, and carrots, then sauté for 8 minutes.
4. Add garlic, tomato, and wine then cook for 2 minutes.
5. Stir in bay leaf, thyme, broth, and red pepper then cook for 30 minutes on a simmer.
6. Add zucchini, mushrooms, parsley, and rice to the soup then continue cooking for 15 minutes.
7. Serve warm with lemon juice on top.

NUTRITION: Calories: 215 Protein: 20 g Carbohydrates: 22 g Fat: 6 g Cholesterol: 24 mg Sodium: 128 mg Potassium: 528 mg Phosphorus: 197 mg Calcium: 54 mg Fiber: 2.4 g

53. Spaghetti Squash & Yellow Bell-Pepper Soup

Preparation time: 10 minutes

Cooking time: 45 minutes

Servings: 4

INGREDIENTS

- 2 diced yellow bell peppers
- 2 chopped large garlic cloves
- 1 peeled and cubed spaghetti squash
- 1 quartered and sliced onion
- 1 tablespoon dried thyme
- 1 tablespoon coconut oil
- 1 teaspoon curry powder
- 4 cups water

DIRECTIONS

1. Heat the oil before sweating the onions and garlic for 3-4 minutes.
2. Sprinkle over the curry powder.
3. Add in the stock and then bring to a boil over a high heat before adding the squash, pepper and thyme.
4. Turn down the heat, cover and allow to simmer for 25-30 minutes.
5. Continue to simmer until squash is soft if needed.
6. Allow to cool before blitzing in a blender/food processor until smooth.
7. Serve!

NUTRITION: Calories 103, Protein 2 g, Carbs 17 g, Fat 4 g, Sodium (Na) 32 mg, Potassium (K)365 mg, Phosphorus 50 mg

54. Red Pepper & Brie Soup

Preparation time: 10 minutes

Cooking time: 35 minutes

Servings: 4

INGREDIENTS

- 1 teaspoon paprika
- 1 teaspoon cumin
- 1 chopped red onion
- 2 chopped garlic cloves
- ¼ cup crumbled brie
- 2 tablespoons. extra virgin olive oil
- 4 chopped red bell peppers
- 4 cups water

DIRECTIONS

1. Sweat in the peppers & onion for 5 minutes.
2. Add the garlic cloves, cumin and paprika and sauté for 3-4 minutes.
3. Add the water and allow to boil before turning the heat down to simmer for 30 minutes.
4. And then remove it from the heat and then allow it to cool slightly.
5. Blend it until smooth after putting the mixture in a food processor.
6. Pour into serving bowls and add the crumbled brie to the top with a little black pepper.
7. Enjoy!

NUTRITION: Calories 152, Protein 3 g, Carbs 8 g, Fat 11 g, Sodium (Na) 66 mg, Potassium (K) 270 mg, Phosphorus 207 mg

55. Turkey & Lemon-Grass Soup

Preparation time: 5 minutes

Cooking time: 40 minutes

Servings: 4

INGREDIENTS

- 1 fresh lime
- ¼ cup fresh basil leaves
- 1 tablespoon cilantro
- 1 cup canned and drained water chestnuts
- 1 tablespoon coconut oil
- 1 thumb-size minced ginger piece
- 2 chopped scallions
- 1 finely chopped green chili
- 4 ounce skinless and sliced turkey breasts
- 1 minced garlic clove, minced
- ½ finely sliced stick lemon-grass
- 1 chopped white onion, chopped
- 4 cups water

DIRECTIONS

1. Crush the lemon-grass, cilantro, chili, 1 tablespoon oil and basil leaves in a blender or pestle and mortar to form a paste.
2. Heat a large pan/wok with 1 tablespoon olive oil on high heat.
3. Sauté the onions, garlic and ginger until soft.
4. Add the turkey and brown each side for 4-5 minutes.
5. Add the broth and stir.
6. Now add the paste and stir.
7. Next add the water chestnuts, turn down the heat slightly and allow to simmer for 25-30 minutes or until turkey is thoroughly cooked through.
8. Serve hot with the green onion sprinkled over the top.

NUTRITION: Calories 123, Protein 10 g, Carbs 12 g, Fat 3 g, Sodium (Na) 501 mg, Potassium (K) 151 mg, Phosphorus 110 mg

56. Paprika Pork Soup

Preparation time: 5 minutes

Cooking time: 35 minutes

Servings: 2

INGREDIENTS

- 4-ounce sliced pork loin
- 1 teaspoon black pepper
- 2 minced garlic cloves
- 1 cup baby spinach
- 3 cups water
- 1 tablespoon extra-virgin olive oil
- 1 chopped onion
- 1 tablespoon paprika

DIRECTIONS

1. Add in the oil, chopped onion and minced garlic.
2. Sauté for 5 minutes on low heat.
3. Add the pork slices to the onions and cook for 7-8 minutes or until browned.
4. Add the water to the pan and bring to a boil on high heat.
5. Stir in the spinach, reduce heat and simmer for a further 20 minutes or until pork is thoroughly cooked through.
6. Season with pepper to serve.

NUTRITION: Calories 165, Protein 13 g, Carbs 10 g, Fat 9 g, Sodium (Na) 269 mg, Potassium (K) 486 mg, Phosphorus 158 mg

57. Mediterranean Vegetable Soup

Preparation time: 5 minutes

Cooking time: 30 minutes

Servings: 4

INGREDIENTS

- 1 tablespoon oregano
- 2 minced garlic cloves
- 1 teaspoon black pepper
- 1 diced zucchini
- 1 cup diced eggplant
- 4 cups water
- 1 diced red pepper
- 1 tablespoon extra-virgin olive oil
- 1 diced red onion

DIRECTIONS

1. Soak the vegetables in warm water prior to use.
2. Add in the oil, chopped onion and minced garlic.
3. Sweat for 5 minutes on low heat.
4. Add the other vegetables to the onions and cook for 7-8 minutes.
5. Add the stock to the pan and bring to a boil on high heat.
6. Stir in the herbs, reduce the heat, and simmer for a further 20 minutes or until thoroughly cooked through.
7. Season with pepper to serve.

NUTRITION: Calories 152, Protein 1 g, Carbs 6 g, Fat 3 g, Sodium (Na) 3 mg, Potassium (K) 229 mg, Phosphorus 45 mg

58. Tofu Soup

Preparation time: 5 minutes

Cooking time: 10 minutes

Servings: 2

INGREDIENTS

- 1 tablespoon miso paste
- 1/8 cup cubed soft tofu
- 1 chopped green onion
- ¼ cup sliced Shiitake mushrooms
- 3 cups Renal stock
- 1 tablespoon soy sauce

DIRECTIONS

1. Take a saucepan, pour the stock into this pan and let it boil on high heat. Reduce heat to medium and let this stock simmer. Add mushrooms in this stock and cook for almost 3 minutes.
2. Take a bowl and mix Soy sauce (reduced salt) and miso paste together in this bowl. Add this mixture and tofu in stock. Simmer for nearly 5 minutes and serve with chopped green onion.

NUTRITION: Calories 129, Fat 7.8g, Sodium (Na) 484mg, Potassium (K) 435mg, Protein 11g, Carbs 5.5g, Phosphorus 73.2mg

59. Onion Soup

Preparation time: 15 minutes

Cooking time: 45 minutes

Servings: 6

INGREDIENTS

- 2 tablespoons. chicken stock
- 1 cup chopped Shiitake mushrooms
- 1 tablespoon minced chives
- 3 teaspoons. beef bouillon
- 1 teaspoon grated ginger root
- ½ chopped carrot
- 1 cup sliced Portobello mushrooms
- 1 chopped onion
- ½ chopped celery stalk
- 2 quarts water
- ¼ teaspoon minced garlic

DIRECTIONS

1. Take a saucepan and combine carrot, onion, celery, garlic, mushrooms (some mushrooms) and ginger in this pan. Add water, beef bouillon and chicken stock in this pan. Put this pot on high heat and let it boil. Decrease flame to medium and cover this pan to cook for almost 45 minutes.
2. Put all remaining mushrooms in one separate pot. Once the boiling mixture is completely done, put one strainer over this new bowl with mushrooms and strain cooked soup in this pot over mushrooms. Discard solid-strained materials.
3. Serve delicious broth with yummy mushrooms in small bowls and sprinkle chives over each bowl.

NUTRITION: Calories 22, Fat 0g, Sodium (Na) 602.3mg, Potassium (K) 54.1mg, Carbs 4.9g, Protein 0.6g, Phosphorus 15.8mg

60. Steakhouse Soup

Preparation Time: 15 minutes

Cooking time: 25 minutes

Servings: 4

INGREDIENTS

- 2 tablespoons. soy sauce
- 2 boneless and cubed chicken breasts.
- ¼ pound halved and trimmed snow peas
- 1 tablespoon minced ginger root
- 1 minced garlic clove
- 1 cup water
- 2 chopped green onions
- 3 cups chicken stock
- 1 chopped carrot
- 3 sliced mushrooms

DIRECTIONS

1. Take a pot and combine ginger, water, chicken stock, Soy sauce (reduced salt) and garlic in this pot. Let them boil on medium heat, mix in chicken pieces, and let them simmer on low heat for almost 15 minutes to tender chicken.
2. Stir in carrot and snow peas and simmer for almost 5 minutes. Add mushrooms in this blend and continue cooking to tender vegetables for nearly 3 minutes. Mix in the chopped onion and serve hot.

NUTRITION: Calories 319, Carbs 14g, Fat 15g, Potassium (K) 225 mg, Protein 29g, Sodium (Na) 389 mg, Phosphorous 190 mg

61. Chinese-style Beef Stew

Preparation Time: 15 minutes

Cooking Time: 6-8 hours

Servings: 6

INGREDIENTS

- 2 medium carrots
- 2 green onions
- 2 celery stalks
- 1 medium green bell pepper, sliced
- 1 garlic clove
- 8 ounce of canned bean sprouts
- 8 ounce of canned water chestnuts
- 2 tablespoon of coconut oil
- 12ounce lean casserole beef, cut into cubes
- ½ cup low-sodium beef stock
- 1 tablespoon brown sugar
- 1/4 cup white wine vinegar
- 1 red chili, finely diced
- 1 ½ cups of water
- 3 cups cooked white rice

DIRECTIONS

1. Slice the carrots, green onions, celery and green pepper.
2. Crush the garlic. (Hint: Use the flat edge of a knife to do this easily.)
3. Rinse and slice the bamboo shoots and water chestnuts.
4. Heat the coconut oil and just brown the beef all over.
5. Transfer the beef to the slow cooker.
6. Add all the ingredients except the water.
7. Stir, it and then cover and cook on Low for 6 to 8 hours.
8. Turn the slow cooker up to High.
9. Add the cold water to the slow cooker.
10. Stir it in to make it smooth, and leave the cooker lid slightly open.
11. Cook for a further 15 minutes.
12. Serve your dish over a bed of rice.

NUTRITION: Per Serving: Calories: 267Protein: 14gCarbohydrates: 31g Fat: 9g Cholesterol: 35mg Sodium: 166mg Potassium: 319mg Phosphorus: 148mg Calcium: 41mg Fiber: 3g

62. Stuffed Bell Pepper Soup

Preparation Time: 5 minutes

Cooking Time: 20 minutes

Servings: 2

INGREDIENTS

- Chicken broth, low-sodium – 2 cups
- Bell pepper, red, diced – 1
- Garlic, minced – 4 cloves
- Onion, diced - .5 cup
- Ground turkey – 4 ounces
- Olive oil – 2 teaspoons
- Italian seasoning – 1 teaspoon
- White rice, cooked – 1 cup
- Parsley, fresh, chopped – 1 tablespoon

DIRECTIONS

1. Cook the ground turkey with the onion, olive oil, , and garlic until the turkey is fully cooked and no pink is remaining about five to seven minutes.
2. Add the black pepper, Italian seasoning, and bell pepper to the soup pot, allowing it to cook for three more minutes.
3. Into the pot, pour the low-sodium chicken broth, simmer the soup for fifteen minutes, until the bell peppers are tender. Stir in the cooked rice and parsley before serving.

NUTRITION: Calories in Individual Servings: 283 Protein Grams: 16 Phosphorus Milligrams: 183 Potassium Milligrams: 369 Sodium Milligrams: 85 Fat Grams: 9 Total Carbohydrates Grams: 32 Net Carbohydrates Grams: 30

63. Salmon Chowder

Preparation time: 20 minutes

Cooking time: 4 hours

Servings: 2

INGREDIENTS

- 3 pounds salmon fillets, sliced into manageable pieces
- 1 1/2 cups onion, chopped
- 2 potatoes, cubed – limit this
- 3 cups water
- 1/3 teaspoon pepper
- 18-ounce evaporated milk, non-fat

DIRECTIONS

1. Put together onion, salmon, potatoes, and pepper in the slow cooker. Pour water
2. Cover and cook for 8 hours on low. Secure the lid.
3. After the 8-hour cooking cycle, turn off the heat. Adjust seasoning according to your preferred taste.
4. Stir in milk. Cover and cook for another 30 minutes. Serve right away.

NUTRITION: Protein: 33.8 g Potassium: 204.3 mg Sodium: 183.5 mg

64. Beef Stew Pasta

Preparation time: 15 minutes

Cooking time: 8 hours

Servings: 2

INGREDIENTS

- 1 Tablespoon olive oil
- 3/4-pound beef round roast, sliced into bite-sized pieces
- 1/2 cup onion, chopped
- 1/2 cup carrots, chopped
- 1/2 cup celery, chopped
- 2 cups beef broth, no salt
- 1/2 teaspoon oregano
- 1/4 cup red wine
- 1/4 teaspoon thyme
- 1/4 teaspoon black pepper
- 2 small tomatoes, diced – limit this
- 1/4 cup whole wheat pasta

DIRECTIONS

1. Pour olive oil into non-stick skillet. Cook beef round roast, in batches, for 5 minutes or until browned all over. Transfer meat to the slow cooker.
2. Add in onion, tomatoes, carrots, celery, beef broth, oregano, red wine, thyme, black pepper, and pasta. Stir mixture well.
3. Cover and cook for 8 to 9 hours on low. Secure the lid.
4. After the 8-hour cooking cycle, turn off the heat. Adjust seasoning according to your preferred taste.
5. To serve, place pasta into plates. Pour sauce all over.

NUTRITION: Protein: 12.8 g Potassium: 128.5mg Sodium: 95.8 mg

65. Italian Chicken Stew

Preparation time: 20 minutes

Cooking time: 8 hours

Servings: 1

INGREDIENTS

- 1/2-pound chicken breast, boneless, skinless, cubed
- 1/3 cup celery, chopped
- 1/2 cup carrot, chopped
- 1/2 cup onion, chopped
- 2 ounce any kind of mushrooms, sliced
- 1/4 teaspoon dill weed
- 1/2 teaspoon Italian seasoning
- 1/4 teaspoon basil
- 1/4 teaspoon black pepper
- 1 tomato, diced – limit this

DIRECTIONS

1. Place chicken breast cubes into the slow cooker.
2. Add in onion, carrot, Italian seasoning, mushrooms, celery, basil, dill weed, and black pepper. Add in diced tomatoes. Mix well.
3. Cover and cook for 8 to 9 hours on low. Secure the lid.
4. After the 8-hour cooking cycle, turn off the heat. Adjust seasoning according to your preferred taste.
5. Serve warm.

NUTRITION: Protein: 29.9 g Potassium: 89.6 mg Sodium: 56.3 mg

66. Turkey Pasta Stew

Preparation time: 10 minutes

Cooking time: 8 hours

Servings: 1

INGREDIENTS

- 1/2-pound ground turkey
- 1/2 cup carrots, sliced
- 1/2 fennel bulb, chopped
- 1/4 cup celery, sliced
- 1 cup chicken broth, low sodium
- 1/3 teaspoon garlic, minced
- 1/2 teaspoon oregano
- 1/2 teaspoon basil
- 1/2 cup shell pasta, uncooked
- 1 cup navy beans, unsalted, cooked

DIRECTIONS

1. Cook turkey in a non-stick skillet set over medium heat until browned on all sides. Transfer to the slow cooker.
2. Add in garlic, carrots, chicken broth, navy beans, basil celery, pasta, oregano, and fennel. Stir well to combine.
3. Cover and cook for 8 to 9 hours on low. Secure the lid.
4. After the 8-hour cooking cycle, turn off the heat. Adjust seasoning according to your preferred taste. Serve warm.

NUTRITION: Protein: 18.8 g Potassium: 84.6 mg Sodium: 68.5 mg

67. One-Pot Chicken Pie Stew

Preparation Time: 15 minutes

Cooking Time: 1 hour 15 minutes

Servings: 8

INGREDIENTS

- Fresh chicken breast (skinless and boneless) – 1½ pounds
- Low-sodium chicken stock – 2 cups
- Canola oil – ¼ cup
- Flour – ½ cup
- Fresh carrots (diced) – ½ cup
- Fresh onions (diced) – ½ cup
- Fresh celery (diced) – ¼ cup
- Black pepper – ½ teaspoon
- Italian seasoning (sodium-free) – 1 tablespoon
- Low-sodium Better Than Bouillon® Chicken Base – 2 teaspoons
- Frozen sweet peas (thawed) – ½ cup
- Heavy cream – ½ cup
- Frozen piecrust (cooked, broken into bite-sized pieces) – 1
- Cheddar cheese (low-fat) – 1 cup

DIRECTIONS

1. Start by pounding the chicken to tenderize it. Cut into small equal-sized cubes.
2. Place it over a medium-high flame. Add in the stock and the chicken. Cook for about 30 minutes.
3. Add in the flour and oil, while the chicken is cooking, mix well to combine.
4. Stir the flour and oil mixture into the broth mixture. Keep stirring until the chicken broth starts to thicken.
5. Reduce the flame to low and cook for another 15 minutes.
6. Now add in the carrots, celery, onions, Italian seasoning, bouillon, and black pepper. Cook for another 15 minutes.
7. Add in the cream and peas after turning off the flame. Keep stirring to mix well.
8. Transfer into soup mugs and top with the cheese and broken pie crust pieces.

NUTRITION: Protein – 26 g Carbohydrates – 22 g Fat – 21 g Cholesterol – 82 mg Sodium – 424 mg Potassium – 209 mg Phosphorus – 290 mg Calcium – 88 mg Fiber – 2 g

FISH AND SEAFOOD

68. Curried Fish Cakes

Preparation Time: 10 minutes

Cooking Time: 18 minutes

Servings: 4

INGREDIENTS

- ¾ pound Atlantic cod, cubed
- 1 apple, peeled and cubed
- 1 tablespoon yellow curry paste
- 2 tablespoons cornstarch
- 1 tablespoon peeled grated ginger root
- 1 large egg
- 1 tablespoon freshly squeezed lemon juice
- ⅛ teaspoon freshly ground black pepper
- ½ cup crushed puffed rice cereal
- 1 tablespoon olive oil

DIRECTIONS

1. Put the cod, apple, curry, cornstarch, ginger, egg, lemon juice, and pepper in a blender or food processor and process until finely chopped. Avoid over-processing, or the mixture will become mushy.
2. Place the rice cereal on a shallow plate.
3. Form the mixture into 8 patties.
4. Dredge the patties in the rice cereal to coat.
5. Cook patties for 3 to 5 minutes per side, turning once until a meat thermometer registers 160°F.
6. Serve.

NUTRITION: Per Serving: Calories: 188; Total fat: 6g; Saturated fat: 1g; Sodium: 150mg; Potassium: 292mg; Phosphorus: 150mg; Carbohydrates: 12g; Fiber: 1g; Protein: 21g; Sugar: 5g

69. Baked Sole with Caramelized Onion

Preparation Time: 10 minutes

Cooking Time: 20 minutes

Servings: 4

INGREDIENTS

- 1 cup finely chopped onion
- ½ cup low-sodium vegetable broth
- 1 yellow summer squash, sliced
- 2 cups frozen broccoli florets
- 4 (3-ounce) fillets of sole
- Pinch salt
- 2 tablespoons olive oil
- Pinch baking soda
- 2 teaspoons avocado oil
- 1 teaspoon dried basil leaves

DIRECTIONS

1. Preheat the oven to 425°F.
2. Add the onions. Cook for 1 minute; then, stirring constantly, cook for another 4 minutes.
3. Remove the onions from the heat.
4. Pour the broth into a baking sheet with a lip and arrange the squash and broccoli on the sheet in a single layer. Top the vegetables with the fish. Sprinkle the fish with the salt and drizzle everything with the olive oil.
5. Bake the fish and the vegetables for 10 minutes.
6. While the fish is baking, return the skillet with the onions to medium-high heat and stir in a pinch of baking soda. Stir in the avocado oil and cook for 5 minutes, stirring frequently, until the onions are dark brown.
7. Transfer the onions to a plate.
8. Tp the fish evenly with the onions. Sprinkle with the basil.
9. Return the fish to the oven, after this bake it 8 to10 minutes Serve the fish on the vegetables.

NUTRITION: Per Serving: Calories: 202; Total fat: 11g; Saturated fat: 3g; Sodium: 320mg; Potassium: 537; Phosphorus: 331mg; Carbohydrates: 10g; Fiber: 3g; Protein: 16g; Sugar: 4g

70. Thai Tuna Wraps

Preparation Time: 10 minutes

Cooking Time: 0 minute

Servings: 4

INGREDIENTS

- ¼ cup unsalted peanut butter
- 2 tablespoons freshly squeezed lemon juice
- 1 teaspoon low-sodium soy sauce
- ½ teaspoon ground ginger
- ⅛ teaspoon cayenne pepper
- 1 (6-ounce) can no-salt-added or low-sodium chunk light tuna, drained
- 1 cup shredded red cabbage
- 2 scallions, white and green parts, chopped
- 1 cup grated carrots
- 8 butter lettuce leaves

DIRECTIONS

1. In a medium bowl, stir together the peanut butter, lemon juice, soy sauce, ginger, and cayenne pepper until well combined.
2. Stir in the tuna, cabbage, scallions, and carrots.

3. Divide the tuna filling evenly between the butter lettuce leaves and serve.

NUTRITION: Per Serving: Calories: 175; Total fat; 10g; Saturated fat: 1g; Sodium: 98mg; Potassium: 421mg; Phosphorus: 153mg; Carbohydrates: 8g; Fiber: 2g; Protein: 17g; Sugar: 4g

71. Grilled Fish and Vegetable Packets

Preparation Time: 15 minutes

Cooking Time: 12 minutes

Servings: 4

INGREDIENTS

- 1 (8-ounce) package sliced mushrooms
- 1 leek, white and green parts, chopped
- 1 cup frozen corn
- 4 (4-ounce) Atlantic cod fillets
- Juice of 1 lemon
- 3 tablespoons olive oil

DIRECTIONS

1. Prepare and preheat the grill to medium coals and set a grill 6 inches from the coals.
2. Tear off four 30-inch long strips of heavy-duty aluminum foil.
3. Arrange the mushrooms, leek, and corn in the center of each piece of foil and top with the fish.
4. Drizzle the packet contents evenly with the lemon juice and olive oil.
5. Bring the longer length sides of the foil together at the top and, holding the edges together, fold them over twice and then fold in the width sides to form a sealed packet with room for the steam.
6. Put the packets on the grill and grill for 10 to 12 minutes until the vegetables are tender-crisp and the fish flakes when tested with a fork. Be careful opening the packets because the escaping steam can be scalding.

NUTRITION: Per Serving: Calories: 267; Total fat: 12g; Saturated fat: 2g; Sodium: 97mg; Potassium: 582mg; Phosphorus: 238mg; Carbohydrates: 13g; Fiber: 2g; Protein: 29g; Sugar: 3g

72. White Fish Soup

Preparation Time: 15 minutes

Cooking Time: 20 minutes

Servings: 4

INGREDIENTS

- 2 tablespoons olive oil
- 1 onion, finely diced
- 1 green bell pepper, chopped
- 1 rib celery, thinly sliced
- 3 cups chicken broth, or more to taste
- 1/4 cup chopped fresh parsley
- 1 1/2 pounds cod, cut into 3/4-inch cubes
- Pepper to taste
- 1 dash red pepper flakes

DIRECTIONS

1. Heat oil in a soup pot over medium heat.
2. Add onion, bell pepper, and celery and cook until wilted, about 5 minutes.
3. Add broth and then bring to a simmer, about 5 minutes.
4. Cook 15 to 20 minutes.
5. Add cod, parsley, and red pepper flakes and simmer until fish flakes easily with a fork, 8 to 10 minutes more.
6. Season with black pepper.

NUTRITION: Calories 117, Total Fat 7.2g, Saturated Fat 1.4g, Cholesterol 18mg, Sodium 37mg, Total Carbohydrate 5.4g, Dietary Fiber 1.3g, Total Sugars 2.8g, Protein 8.1g, Calcium 23mg, Iron 1mg, Potassium 122mg, Phosphorus 111 mg

73. Lemon Butter Salmon

Preparation Time: 15 minutes

Cooking Time: 15 minutes

Servings: 6

INGREDIENTS

- 1 tablespoon butter
- 2 tablespoons olive oil
- 1 tablespoon Dijon mustard
- 1 tablespoons lemon juice
- 2 cloves garlic, crushed
- 1 teaspoon dried dill
- 1 teaspoon dried basil leaves
- 1 tablespoon capers
- 24-ounce salmon filet

DIRECTIONS

1. Put all of the ingredients except the salmon in a saucepan over medium heat.
2. Bring to a boil and then simmer for 5 minutes.
3. Preheat your grill.
4. Create a packet using foil.
5. Place the sauce and salmon inside.
6. Seal the packet.
7. Grill for 12 minutes.

NUTRITION: Calories 292 Protein 22 g Carbohydrates 2 g Fat 22 g Cholesterol 68 mg Sodium 190 mg Potassium 439 mg Phosphorus 280 mg Calcium 21 mg

74. Crab Cake

Preparation Time: 15 minutes

Cooking Time: 9 minutes

Servings: 6

INGREDIENTS

- 1/4 cup onion, chopped
- 1/4 cup bell pepper, chopped
- 1 egg, beaten
- 6 low-sodium crackers, crushed
- 1/4 cup low-fat mayonnaise
- 1-pound crab meat
- 1 tablespoon dry mustard
- Pepper to taste
- 2 tablespoons lemon juice
- 1 tablespoon fresh parsley
- 1 tablespoon garlic powder
- 3 tablespoons olive oil

DIRECTIONS

1. Mix all the ingredients except the oil.
2. Form 6 patties from the mixture.
3. Pour the oil into a pan in a medium heat.
4. Cook the crab cakes for 5 minutes.
5. Flip and cook for another 4 minutes.

NUTRITION: Calories 189 Protein 13 g Carbohydrates 5 g Fat 14 g Cholesterol 111 mg Sodium 342 mg Potassium 317 mg Phosphorus 185 mg Calcium 52 mg Fiber 0.5 g

75. Baked Fish in Cream Sauce

Preparation Time: 10 minutes

Cooking Time: 40 minutes

Servings: 4

INGREDIENTS

- 1-pound haddock
- 1/2 cup all-purpose flour
- 2 tablespoons butter (unsalted)
- 1/4 teaspoon pepper
- 2 cups fat-free nondairy creamer
- 1/4 cup water

DIRECTIONS

1. Preheat your oven to 350 degrees F.
2. Spray baking pan with oil.
3. Sprinkle with a little flour.
4. Arrange fish on the pan
5. Season with pepper.
6. Sprinkle remaining flour on the fish.
7. Spread creamer on both sides of the fish.
8. Bake for 40 minutes or until golden.
9. Spread cream sauce on top of the fish before serving.

NUTRITION: Calories 383 Protein 24 g Carbohydrates 46 g Fat 11 g Cholesterol 79 mg Sodium 253 mg Potassium 400 mg Phosphorus 266 mg Calcium 46 mg Fiber 0.4 g

76. Shrimp & Broccoli

Preparation Time: 10 minutes

Cooking Time: 5 minutes

Servings: 4

INGREDIENTS

- 1 tablespoon olive oil
- 1 clove garlic, minced
- 1-pound shrimp
- 1/4 cup red bell pepper
- 1 cup broccoli florets, steamed
- 10-ounce cream cheese
- 1/2 teaspoon garlic powder
- 1/4 cup lemon juice
- 3/4 teaspoon ground peppercorns
- 1/4 cup half and half creamer

DIRECTIONS

1. Pour the oil and cook garlic for 30 seconds.
2. Add shrimp and cook for 2 minutes.
3. Add the rest of the ingredients.
4. Mix well.
5. Cook for 2 minutes.

NUTRITION: Calories 469 Protein 28 g Carbohydrates 28 g Fat 28 g Cholesterol 213 mg Sodium 374 mg Potassium 469 mg Phosphorus 335 mg Calcium 157 mg Fiber 2.6 g

77. Shrimp in Garlic Sauce

Preparation Time: 10 minutes

Cooking Time: 6 minutes

Servings: 4

INGREDIENTS

- 3 tablespoons butter (unsalted)
- 1/4 cup onion, minced
- 3 cloves garlic, minced
- 1-pound shrimp, shelled and deveined
- 1/2 cup half and half creamer
- 1/4 cup white wine
- 2 tablespoons fresh basil
- Black pepper to taste

DIRECTIONS

1. Add butter to a pan over medium low heat.
2. Let it melt.
3. Add the onion and garlic.
4. Cook for it 1-2 minutes.

5. Add the shrimp and cook for 2 minutes.
6. Transfer shrimp on a serving platter and set aside.
7. Add the rest of the ingredients.
8. Simmer for 3 minutes.
9. Pour sauce over the shrimp and serve.

NUTRITION: Calories 482 Protein 33 g Carbohydrates 46 g Fat 11 g Cholesterol 230 mg Sodium 213 mg Potassium 514 mg Phosphorus 398 mg Calcium 133 mg Fiber 2.0 g

78. Fish Taco

Preparation Time: 40 minutes

Cooking Time: 10 minutes

Servings: 6

INGREDIENTS

- 1 tablespoon lime juice
- 1 tablespoon olive oil
- 1 clove garlic, minced
- 1-pound cod fillets
- 1/2 teaspoon ground cumin
- 1/4 teaspoon black pepper
- 1/2 teaspoon chili powder
- 1/4 cup sour cream
- 1/2 cup mayonnaise
- 2 tablespoons nondairy milk
- 1 cup cabbage, shredded
- 1/2 cup onion, chopped
- 1/2 bunch cilantro, chopped
- 12 corn tortillas

DIRECTIONS

1. Drizzle lemon juice over the fish fillet.
2. And then coat it with olive oil and then season with garlic, cumin, pepper and chili powder.
3. Let it sit for 30 minutes.
4. Broil fish for 10 minutes, flipping halfway through.
5. Flake the fish using a fork.
6. In a bowl, mix sour cream, milk and mayo.
7. Assemble tacos by filling each tortilla with mayo mixture, cabbage, onion, cilantro and fish flakes.

NUTRITION: Calories 366 Protein 18 g Carbohydrates 31 g Fat 19 g Cholesterol 40 mg Sodium 194 mg Potassium 507 mg Phosphorus 327 mg Calcium 138 mg Fiber 4.3 g

79. Baked Trout

Preparation Time: 5 minutes

Cooking Time: 10 minutes

Servings: 8

INGREDIENTS

- 2-pound trout fillet
- 1 tablespoon oil
- 1 teaspoon salt-free lemon pepper
- 1/2 teaspoon paprika

DIRECTIONS

1. Preheat your oven to 350 degrees F.
2. Coat fillet with oil.
3. Place fish on a baking pan.
4. Season with lemon pepper and paprika.
5. Bake for 10 minutes.

NUTRITION: Calories 161 Protein 21 g Carbohydrates 0 g Fat 8 g Cholesterol 58 mg Sodium 109 mg Potassium 385 mg Phosphorus 227 mg Calcium 75 mg Fiber 0.1 g

80. Fish with Mushrooms

Preparation Time: 5 minutes

Cooking Time: 16 minutes

Servings: 4

INGREDIENTS

- 1-pound cod fillet
- 2 tablespoons butter
- ¼ cup white onion, chopped
- 1 cup fresh mushrooms
- 1 teaspoon dried thyme

DIRECTIONS

1. Put the fish in a baking pan.
2. Preheat your oven to 450 degrees F.
3. Melt the butter and cook onion and mushroom for 1 minute.
4. Spread mushroom mixture on top of the fish.
5. Season with thyme.
6. Bake in the oven for 15 minutes.

NUTRITION: Calories 156 Protein 21 g Carbohydrates 3 g Fat 7 g Cholesterol 49 mg Sodium 110 mg Potassium 561 mg Phosphorus 225 mg Calcium 30 mg Fiber 0.5 g

81. Salmon with Spicy Honey

Preparation Time: 15 Minutes

Cooking time: 8 minutes

Servings: 2

INGREDIENTS

- 16-ounce salmon fillet
- 3 tablespoon honey
- 3/4 teaspoon lemon peel
- 3 bowls arugula salad
- 1/2 teaspoon black pepper
- 1/2 teaspoon garlic powder
- 2 teaspoon olive oil
- 1 teaspoon hot water

DIRECTIONS

1. Prepare a small bowl with some hot water and put in honey, grated lemon peel, ground pepper, and garlic powder.
2. Spread the mixture over salmon fillets.
3. Warm some olive oil at a medium heat and add spiced salmon fillet and cook for 4 minutes.
4. Turn the fillets on one side then on the other side.
5. Continue to cook for other 4 minutes at a reduced heat and try to check when the salmon fillets flake easily.
6. Put some arugula on each plate and add the salmon fillets on top, adding some aromatic herbs or some dill. Serve and enjoy!

NUTRITION: Calories: 320 Protein: 23 g Sodium: 65 mg Potassium: 450 mg Phosphorus: 250 mg

82. Salmon with Maple Glaze

Preparation Time: 15 minutes

Cooking Time: 2 hours

Servings: 4

INGREDIENTS

- 1-pound salmon fillets
- 1 tablespoon green onion, chopped
- 1 tablespoon low sodium soy sauce
- 2 garlic cloves, pressed
- 2 tablespoon fresh cilantro
- 3 tablespoon lemon juice (or juice of 1 lemon)
- 3 tablespoon maple syrup

DIRECTIONS

1. Combine all ingredients except for salmon.
2. Put salmon on platter and then pour marinade over fillets. Let it marinate 2 hours or more.
3. Preheat broiler.
4. Remove salmon from marinade.
5. Place salmon on bottom rack and broil for 10 minutes. Do not turn over.
6. Serve hot/cold with a wedge of lemon.

NUTRITION: Calories per Serving: 220; carbs: 12g; protein: 24g; fats: 8g; phosphorus: 374mg; potassium: 440mg; sodium: 621mg

83. Steamed Spicy Tilapia Fillet

Preparation Time: 10 minutes

Cooking Time: 25 minutes

Servings: 4

INGREDIENTS

- 4 fillets of tilapia
- 1 teaspoon hot pepper sauce
- 1 large sprig thyme
- 1 tablespoon Ketchup
- 1 tablespoon lime juice
- 1 cup hot water
- 1/2 cup onion, sliced
- 1/4 teaspoon black pepper
- 3/4 cup red and green peppers, sliced

DIRECTIONS

1. In a large shallow dish that fits your steamer, mix well hot pepper sauce, thyme, ketchup, lemon juice, and black pepper. Mix thoroughly.
2. Add tilapia fillets and spoon over sauce.
3. Mix in remaining ingredients except for water. Mix well in sauce.
4. Cover top of dish with foil.
5. Add the hot water in the steamer. Place dish on steamer rack. Cover pot and steam fish and veggies for 20 minutes.
6. Let it stand for 5-6 minutes before serving.

NUTRITION: Calories per Serving: 131; carbs: 5g; protein: 24g; fats: 3g; phosphorus: 212mg; potassium: 457mg; sodium: 102mg

84. Dijon Mustard and Lime Marinated Shrimp

Preparation Time: 20 minutes

Cooking Time: 80 minutes

Servings: 8

INGREDIENTS

- 1-pound uncooked shrimp, peeled and deveined
- 1 bay leaf
- 3 whole cloves
- ½ cup rice vinegar
- 1 cup water
- ½ teaspoon hot sauce

- 2 tablespoons. capers
- 2 tablespoons. Dijon mustard
- ½ cup fresh lime juice, plus lime zest as garnish
- 1 medium red onion, chopped

DIRECTIONS

1. Mix hot sauce, mustard, capers, lime juice and onion in a shallow baking dish and set aside.
2. Bring it to a boil in a large saucepan bay leaf, cloves, vinegar and water.
3. Once boiling, add shrimps and cook for a minute while stirring continuously.
4. Drain shrimps and pour shrimps into onion mixture.
5. For an hour, refrigerate while covered the shrimps.
6. Then serve shrimps cold and garnished with lime zest.

NUTRITION: Calories per Serving: 123; carbs: 3g; protein: 12g; fats: 1g; phosphorus: 119mg; potassium: 87mg; sodium: 568mg

85. Baked Cod Crusted with Herbs

Preparation Time: 15 minutes

Cooking Time: 10 minutes

Servings: 4

INGREDIENTS

- ¼ cup honey
- ½ cup panko
- ½ teaspoon pepper
- 1 tablespoon extra-virgin olive oil
- 1 tablespoon lemon juice
- 1 teaspoon dried basil
- 1 teaspoon dried parsley
- 1 teaspoon rosemary
- 4 pieces of 4-ounce cod fillets

DIRECTIONS

1. With olive oil, grease a 9 x 13-inch baking pan and preheat oven to 375oF.
2. In a zip top bag mix panko, rosemary, pepper, parsley and basil.
3. Evenly spread cod fillets in prepped dish and drizzle with lemon juice.
4. Then brush the fillets with honey on all sides. Discard remaining honey if any.
5. Then evenly divide the panko mixture on top of cod fillets.
6. Pop in the oven and bake for ten minutes or until fish is cooked.
7. Serve and enjoy.

NUTRITION: Calories per Serving: 113; carbs: 21g; protein: 5g; fats: 2g; phosphorus: 89mg; potassium: 115mg; sodium: 139mg

86. Dill Relish on White Sea Bass

Preparation Time: 15 minutes

Cooking Time: 60 minutes

Servings: 4

INGREDIENTS

- 1 lemon, quartered
- 4 pieces of 4-ounce white sea bass fillets
- 1 teaspoon lemon juice
- 1 teaspoon Dijon mustard
- 1 ½ teaspoons. chopped fresh dill
- 1 teaspoon pickled baby capers, drained
- 1 ½ tablespoons. chopped white onion

DIRECTIONS

1. Preheat oven to 375oF.
2. Mix lemon juice, mustard, dill, capers and onions in a small bowl.
3. Prepare four aluminum foil squares and place 1 fillet per foil.
4. Squeeze a lemon wedge per fish.
5. Evenly divide into 4 the dill spread and drizzle over fillet.
6. Close the foil over the fish securely and pop in the oven.
7. Bake for 9 to 12 minutes or until fish is cooked through.
8. Remove from foil and transfer to a serving platter, serve and enjoy.

NUTRITION: Calories per Serving: 71; carbs: 11g; protein: 7g; fats: 1g; phosphorus: 91mg; potassium: 237mg; sodium: 94mg

87. Tilapia with Lemon Garlic Sauce

Preparation Time: 15 minutes

Cooking Time: 30 minutes

Servings: 4

INGREDIENTS

- Pepper
- 1 teaspoon dried parsley flakes
- 1 clove garlic (finely chopped)
- 1 tablespoon butter (melted)
- 3 tablespoons. fresh lemon juice
- 4 tilapia fillets

DIRECTIONS

1. First, spray baking dish with non-stick cooking spray then preheat oven at 375 degrees Fahrenheit (190oC).

In cool water, rinse tilapia fillets and using paper towels pat dry the fillets.

2. Place tilapia fillets in the baking dish then pour butter and lemon juice and top off with pepper, parsley and garlic.
3. Bake tilapia in the preheated oven for 30 minutes and wait until fish is white.
4. Enjoy!

NUTRITION: Calories per Serving: 168; carbs: 4g; protein: 24g; fats: 5g; phosphorus: 207mg; potassium: 431mg; sodium: 85mg

88. Spinach with Tuscan White Beans and Shrimps

Preparation Time: 5 minutes

Cooking Time: 15 minutes

Servings: 4

INGREDIENTS

- 1 ½ ounces crumbled reduce-fat feta cheese
- 5 cups baby spinach
- 15 ounces can no salt added cannellini beans (rinsed and drained)
- ½ cup low sodium, fat-free chicken broth
- 2 tablespoons. balsamic vinegar
- 2 teaspoons. chopped fresh sage
- 4 cloves garlic (minced)
- 1 medium onion (chopped)
- 1-pound large shrimp (peeled and deveined)
- 2 tablespoons. olive oil

DIRECTIONS

1. Heat 1 teaspoon oil. Heat it over medium-high.
2. Then for about 2 to 3 minutes, cook the shrimps using the heated skillet then place them on a plate. Heat on the same skillet the sage, garlic, and onions then cook for about 4 minutes. Add and stir in vinegar for 30 seconds.
3. For about 2 minutes, add chicken broth. Then, add spinach and beans and cook for an additional 2 to 3 minutes.
4. Remove skillet then add and stir in cooked shrimps topped with feta cheese.
5. Serve and divide into 4 bowls. Enjoy!

NUTRITION: Calories per Serving: 343; carbs: 21g; protein: 22g; fats: 11g; phosphorus: 400mg; potassium: 599mg; sodium: 766mg

89. Bagel with Salmon and Egg

Preparation Time: 15 minutes

Cooking Time: 10 minutes

Servings: 1

INGREDIENTS

- Bagel – ½
- Cream cheese – 1 tablespoon
- Scallions – 1 tablespoon
- Fresh dill – ½ teaspoon
- Fresh basil leaves – 2
- Tomato – 1 slice
- Arugula – 4 pieces
- Egg – 1 large
- Cooked salmon – 1 ounce

DIRECTIONS

1. Start by slicing the bagel through the center horizontally. Take one half of the bagel and toast it in an oven or a toaster.
2. Finely chop the dill, basil leaves, and scallions. Set aside.
3. Add in the cream cheese. Toss in the chopped dill, basil, and scallions. Mix well to combine. Take the toasted bagel and spread the herbs and cream cheese mixture evenly over it.
4. Place the tomato slice and arugula on top. Set aside.
5. Take a small mixing bowl and then beat the egg.
6. Take a non-stick saucepan and grease it using cooking spray. Stir after pouring the beaten egg into the pan and. Cook for about 1 minute over medium heat. Keep stirring to make a perfect scrambled egg.
7. Take the cooked salmon and place it in the same pan as the egg. This will help you heat the salmon and cook the egg at the same time.
8. Place the scrambled egg over the tomato slice and top it with the salmon.

NUTRITION: Protein – 19 g Fat – 14 g Carbohydrates – 29 g Cholesterol – 218 mg Potassium – 338 mg Sodium – 378 mg Phosphorus – 270 mg Fiber – 2.6 g Calcium – 77 m

90. Salmon Stuffed Pasta

Preparation time: 20 minutes

Cooking time: 35 minutes

Servings: 24

INGREDIENTS:

- 24 jumbo pasta shells, boiled
- 1 cup coffee creamer
- Filling:
- 2 eggs, beaten
- 2 cups creamed cottage cheese
- ¼ cup chopped onion
- 1 red bell pepper, diced
- 2 teaspoons dried parsley
- ½ teaspoon lemon peel
- 1 can salmon, drained
- Dill Sauce:
- 1 ½ teaspoon butter
- 1 ½ teaspoon flour
- 1/8 teaspoon pepper
- 1 tablespoon lemon juice
- 1 ½ cup coffee creamer
- 2 teaspoons dried dill weed

DIRECTION:

1. Beat the cream cheese with the egg and all the other filling ingredients in a bowl.
2. Divide the filling in the pasta shells and place the shells in a 9x13 baking dish.
3. Pour the coffee creamer around the stuffed shells then cover with a foil.
4. Bake the shells for 30 minutes at 350 degrees F.
5. Meanwhile, whisk all the ingredients for dill sauce in a saucepan.
6. Stir for 5 minutes until it thickens.
7. Pour this sauce over the baked pasta shells.
8. Serve warm.

NUTRITION: Calories 268 Total Fat 4.8g Sodium 86mg Protein 11.5g Calcium 27mg Phosphorous 314mg Potassium 181mg

91. Herbed Vegetable Trout

Preparation time: 15 minutes

Cooking time: 15 minutes

Servings: 4

INGREDIENTS:

- 14 oz. trout fillets
- 1/2 teaspoon herb seasoning blend
- 1 lemon, sliced
- 2 green onions, sliced
- 1 stalk celery, chopped
- 1 medium carrot, julienne

DIRECTION:

1. Prepare and preheat a charcoal grill over moderate heat.
2. Place the trout fillets over a large piece of foil and drizzle herb seasoning on top.
3. Spread the lemon slices, carrots, celery, and green onions over the fish.
4. Cover the fish with foil and pack it.
5. Place the packed fish in the grill and cook for 15 minutes.
6. Once done, remove the foil from the fish.
7. Serve.

NUTRITION: Calories 202 Total Fat 8.5g Sodium 82mg Calcium 70mg Phosphorous 287mg Potassium 560mg

92. Citrus Glazed Salmon

Preparation time: 20 minutes

Cooking time: 17 minutes

Servings: 4

INGREDIENTS:

- 2 garlic cloves, crushed
- 1 1/2 tablespoons lemon juice
- 2 tablespoons olive oil
- 1 tablespoon butter
- 1 tablespoon Dijon mustard
- 2 dashes cayenne pepper
- 1 teaspoon dried basil leaves
- 1 teaspoon dried dill
- 24 oz. salmon filet

DIRECTION:

1. Place a 1-quart saucepan over moderate heat and add the oil, butter, garlic, lemon juice, mustard, cayenne pepper, dill, and basil to the pan.
2. Stir this mixture for 5 minutes after it has boiled.
3. Prepare and preheat a charcoal grill over moderate heat.
4. Place the fish on a foil sheet and fold the edges to make a foil tray.
5. Pour the prepared sauce over the fish.
6. Place the fish in the foil in the preheated grill and cook for 12 minutes.
7. Slice and serve.

NUTRITION: Calories 401 Total Fat 20.5g Cholesterol 144mg Sodium 256mg Carbohydrate 0.5g Calcium 549mg Phosphorous 214mg Potassium 446mg

93. Broiled Salmon Fillets

Preparation time: 10 minutes

Cooking time: 13 minutes

Servings: 4

INGREDIENTS:

- 1 tablespoon ginger root, grated
- 1 clove garlic, minced
- ¼ cup maple syrup
- 1 tablespoon hot pepper sauce
- 4 salmon fillets, skinless

DIRECTION:

1. Grease a pan with cooking spray and place it over moderate heat.
2. Add the ginger and garlic and sauté for 3 minutes then transfer to a bowl.
3. Add the hot pepper sauce and maple syrup to the ginger-garlic.
4. Mix well and keep this mixture aside.
5. Place the salmon fillet in a suitable baking tray, greased with cooking oil.
6. Brush the maple sauce over the fillets liberally
7. Broil them for 10 minutes at the oven at broiler settings.
8. Serve warm.

NUTRITION: Calories 289 Total Fat 11.1g Sodium 80mg Carbohydrate 13.6g Calcium 78mg Phosphorous 230mg Potassium 331mg

94. Broiled Shrimp

Preparation time: 10 minutes

Cooking time: 5 minutes

Servings: 8

INGREDIENTS:

- 1 lb. shrimp in shell
- 1/2 cup unsalted butter, melted
- 2 teaspoons lemon juice
- 2 tablespoons chopped onion
- 1 clove garlic, minced
- 1/8 teaspoon pepper

DIRECTION:

1. Toss the shrimp with the butter, lemon juice, onion, garlic, and pepper in a bowl.
2. Spread the seasoned shrimp in a baking tray.
3. Broil for 5 minutes in an oven on broiler setting.
4. Serve warm.

NUTRITION: Calories 164 Total Fat 12.8g Sodium 242mg Carbohydrate 0.6g Calcium 45mg Phosphorous 215mg Potassium 228mg

95. Grilled Lemony Cod

Preparation time: 10 minutes

Cooking time: 10 minutes

Servings: 4

INGREDIENTS:

- 1 lb. cod fillets
- 1 teaspoon salt-free lemon pepper seasoning
- 1/4 cup lemon juice

DIRECTION:

1. Rub the cod fillets with lemon pepper seasoning and lemon juice.
2. Grease a baking tray with cooking spray and place the salmon in the baking tray.
3. Bake the fish for 10 minutes at 350 degrees F in a preheated oven.
4. Serve warm.

NUTRITION: Calories 155 Total Fat 7.1g Cholesterol 50mg Sodium 53mg Protein 22.2g Calcium 43mg Phosphorous 237mg Potassium 461mg

96. Spiced Honey Salmon

Preparation time: 15 minutes

Cooking time: 16 minutes

Servings: 4

INGREDIENTS:

- 3 tablespoons honey
- 3/4 teaspoon lemon peel
- 1/2 teaspoon black pepper
- 1/2 teaspoon garlic powder
- 1 teaspoon water
- 16 oz. salmon fillets
- 2 tablespoons olive oil
- Dill, chopped, to serve

DIRECTION:

1. Whisk the lemon peel with honey, garlic powder, hot water, and ground pepper in a small bowl.
2. Rub this honey mixture over the salmon fillet liberally.
3. Set a suitable skillet over moderate heat and add olive oil to heat.
4. Set the spiced salmon fillets in the pan and sear them for 4 minutes per side.
5. Garnish with dill.
6. Serve warm.

NUTRITION: Calories 264 Total Fat 14.1g Cholesterol 50mg Sodium 55mg Calcium 67mg Phosphorous 174mg Potassium 507mg

VEGETARIAN

97. Tofu Stir Fry

Preparation Time: 15 minutes

Cooking Time: 20 minutes

Servings: 4

INGREDIENTS

- 1 teaspoon sugar
- 1 tablespoon lime juice
- 1 tablespoon low sodium soy sauce
- 2 tablespoons cornstarch
- 2 egg whites, beaten
- 1/2 cup unseasoned bread crumbs
- 1 tablespoon vegetable oil
- 16 ounces tofu, cubed
- 1 clove garlic, minced
- 1 tablespoon sesame oil
- 1 red bell pepper, sliced into strips
- 1 cup broccoli florets
- 1 teaspoon herb seasoning blend
- Dash black pepper
- Sesame seeds
- Steamed white rice

DIRECTIONS

1. Dissolve sugar in a mixture of lime juice and soy sauce. Set aside.
2. In the first bowl, put the cornstarch.
3. Add the egg whites in the second bowl.
4. Place the breadcrumbs in the third bowl.
5. Dip each tofu cubes in the first, second and third bowls.
6. Pour vegetable oil in a pan over medium heat.
7. Cook tofu cubes until golden.
8. Drain the tofu and set aside.
9. Remove oil from the pan and add sesame oil.
10. Add garlic, bell pepper and broccoli.
11. Cook until crisp tender.
12. Season with the seasoning blend and pepper.
13. Put the tofu back and toss to mix.
14. Pour soy sauce mixture on top and transfer to serving bowls.
15. Garnish with the sesame seeds and serve on top of white rice.

NUTRITION: Calories 401 Protein 19 g Carbohydrates 46 g Fat 16 g Cholesterol 0 mg Sodium 584 mg Potassium 317 mg Phosphorus 177 mg Calcium 253 mg Fiber 2.7 g

98. Broccoli Pancake

Preparation Time: 10 minutes

Cooking Time: 5 minutes

Servings: 4

INGREDIENTS

- 3 cups broccoli florets, diced
- 2 eggs, beaten
- 2 tablespoons all-purpose flour
- 1/2 cup onion, chopped
- 2 tablespoons olive oil

DIRECTIONS

1. Boil broccoli in water for 5 minutes. Drain and set aside.
2. Mix egg and flour.
3. Add onion and broccoli to the mixture.
4. Cook the broccoli pancake until brown on both sides.

NUTRITION: Calories 140 Protein 6 g Carbohydrates 7 g Fat 10 g Cholesterol 106 mg Sodium 58 mg Potassium 276 mg Phosphorus 101 mg Calcium 50 mg Fiber 2.1 g

99. Carrot Casserole

Preparation Time: 10 minutes

Cooking Time: 20 minutes

Serving: 8

INGREDIENTS

- 1-pound carrots, sliced into rounds
- 12 low-sodium crackers
- 2 tablespoons butter
- 2 tablespoons onion, chopped
- 1/4 cup cheddar cheese, shredded

DIRECTIONS

1. Preheat your oven to 350 degrees F.
2. Boil carrots in a pot of water until tender.
3. Drain the carrots and reserve ¼ cup liquid.
4. Mash carrots.
5. Add all the ingredients into the carrots except cheese.
6. Place the mashed carrots in a casserole dish.
7. Sprinkle cheese on top and bake in the oven for 15 minutes.

NUTRITION: Calories 97 Protein 2 g Carbohydrates 9 g Fat 7 g Cholesterol 13 mg Sodium 174 mg Potassium 153 mg Phosphorus 47 mg Calcium 66 mg Fiber 1.8 g

100. Cauliflower Rice

Preparation Time: 10 minutes

Cooking Time: 10 minutes

Servings: 4

INGREDIENTS

- 1 head cauliflower, sliced into florets
- 1 tablespoon butter
- Black pepper to taste
- 1/4 teaspoon garlic powder
- 1/4 teaspoon herb seasoning blend

DIRECTIONS

1. Put cauliflower florets in a food processor.
2. Pulse until consistency is similar to grain.
3. In a pan over medium heat, melt the butter and add the spices.
4. Toss cauliflower rice and cook for 10 minutes.
5. Fluff using a fork before serving.

NUTRITION: Calories 47 Protein 1 g Carbohydrates 4 g Fat 3 g Cholesterol 8 mg Sodium 43 mg Potassium 206 mg Phosphorus 31 mg Calcium 16 mg Fiber 1.4 g

101. Eggplant Fries

Preparation Time: 10 minutes

Cooking Time: 5 minutes

Servings: 6

INGREDIENTS

- 2 eggs, beaten
- 1 cup almond milk
- 1 teaspoon hot sauce
- 3/4 cup cornstarch
- 3 teaspoons dry ranch seasoning mix
- 3/4 cup dry bread crumbs
- 1 eggplant, sliced into strips
- 1/2 cup oil

DIRECTIONS

1. In a bowl, mix eggs, milk and hot sauce.
2. In a dish, mix cornstarch, seasoning and breadcrumbs.
3. Dip first the eggplant strips in the egg mixture.
4. Coat each strip with the cornstarch mixture.
5. Pour oil in a pan over medium heat.
6. Once hot, add the fries and cook for 3 minutes or until golden.

NUTRITION: Calories 234 Protein 7 g Carbohydrates 25 g Fat 13 g Cholesterol 48 mg Sodium 212 mg Potassium 215 mg Phosphorus 86 mg Calcium 70 mg Fiber 2.1 g

102. Seasoned Green Beans

Preparation Time: 10 minutes

Cooking Time: 10 minutes

Servings: 4

INGREDIENTS

- 10-ounce green beans
- 4 teaspoons butter
- 1/4 cup onion, chopped
- 1/2 cup red bell pepper, chopped
- 1 teaspoon dried dill weed
- 1 teaspoon dried parsley
- 1/4 teaspoon black pepper

DIRECTIONS

1. Boil green beans in a pot of water. Drain.
2. In a pan over medium heat, melt the butter and cook onion and bell pepper.
3. Season with dill and parsley.
4. Put the green beans back to the skillet.
5. Sprinkle pepper on top before serving.

NUTRITION: Calories 67 Protein 2 g Carbohydrates 8 g Fat 3 g Cholesterol 0 mg Sodium 55 mg Potassium 194 mg Phosphorus 32 mg Calcium 68 mg Fiber 4.0 g

103. Grilled Squash

Preparation Time: 10 minutes

Cooking Time: 6 minutes

Servings: 8

INGREDIENTS

- 4 zucchinis, rinsed, drained and sliced
- 4 crookneck squash, rinsed, drained and sliced
- Cooking spray
- 1/4 teaspoon garlic powder
- 1/4 teaspoon black pepper

DIRECTIONS

1. Arrange squash on a baking sheet.
2. Spray with oil.
3. Season with garlic powder and pepper.
4. Grill for 3 minutes per side or until tender but not too soft.

NUTRITION: Calories 17 Protein 1 g Carbohydrates 3 g Fat 0 g Cholesterol 0 mg Sodium 6 mg Potassium 262 mg Phosphorus 39 mg Calcium 16 mg Fiber 1.1 g

105. Thai Tofu Broth

Preparation time: 5 minutes

Cooking time: 15 minutes

Servings: 4

INGREDIENTS

- 1 cup rice noodles
- ½ sliced onion
- 6 ounce drained, pressed and cubed tofu
- ¼ cup sliced scallions
- ½ cup water
- ½ cup canned water chestnuts
- ½ cup rice milk
- 1 tablespoon lime juice
- 1 tablespoon coconut oil
- ½ finely sliced chili
- 1 cup snow peas

DIRECTIONS

1. Heat the oil in a wok on a high heat and then sauté the tofu until brown on each side.
2. Add the onion and sauté for 2-3 minutes.
3. Add the rice milk and water to the wok until bubbling.
4. Lower to medium heat and add the noodles, chili and water chestnuts.
5. Allow to simmer for 10-15 minutes and then add the sugar snap peas for 5 minutes.
6. Serve with a sprinkle of scallions.

NUTRITION: Calories 304, Protein 9 g, Carbs 38 g, Fat 13 g, Sodium (Na) 36 mg, Potassium (K) 114 mg, Phosphorus 101 mg

106. Delicious Vegetarian Lasagna

Preparation time: 10 minutes

Cooking time: 1 hour

Servings: 4

INGREDIENTS

- 1 teaspoon basil
- 1 tablespoon olive oil
- ½ sliced red pepper
- 3 lasagna sheets
- ½ diced red onion
- ¼ teaspoon black pepper
- 1 cup rice milk
- 1 minced garlic clove
- 1 cup sliced eggplant
- ½ sliced zucchini
- ½ pack soft tofu
- 1 teaspoon oregano

DIRECTIONS

1. Preheat oven to 325°F/Gas Mark 3.
2. Slice zucchini, eggplant and pepper into vertical strips.
3. Add the rice milk and tofu to a food processor and blitz until smooth. Set aside.
4. Heat the oil in a skillet over medium heat and add the onions and garlic for 3-4 minutes or until soft.
5. Sprinkle in the herbs and pepper and allow to stir through for 5-6 minutes until hot.
6. Into a lasagna or suitable oven dish, layer 1 lasagna sheet, then 1/3 the eggplant, followed by 1/3 zucchini, then 1/3 pepper before pouring over 1/3 of tofu white sauce.
7. Repeat for the next 2 layers, finishing with the white sauce.
8. Add to the oven for 40-50 minutes or until veg is soft and can easily be sliced into servings.

NUTRITION: Calories 235, Protein 5 g, Carbs 10g, Fat 9 g, Sodium (Na) 35 mg, Potassium (K) 129 mg, Phosphorus 66 mg

107. Chili Tofu Noodles

Preparation time: 5 minutes

Cooking Time: 15 minutes

Servings: 4

INGREDIENTS

- ½ diced red chili
- 2 cups rice noodles
- ½ juiced lime
- 6 ounce pressed and cubed silken firm tofu
- 1 teaspoon grated fresh ginger
- 1 tablespoon coconut oil
- 1 cup green beans
- 1 minced garlic clove

DIRECTIONS

1. Steam the green beans for 10-12 minutes or according to package directions and drain.
2. Cook the noodles in a pot of boiling water for 10-15 minutes or according to package directions.
3. Meanwhile, heat a wok or skillet on a high heat and add coconut oil.
4. Now add the tofu, chili flakes, garlic and ginger and sauté for 5-10 minutes.
5. After doing that, drain in the noodles along with the green beans and lime juice then add it to the wok.
6. Toss to coat.
7. Serve hot!

NUTRITION: Calories 246, Protein 10 g, Carbs 28g, Fat 12 g, Sodium (Na) 25 mg, Potassium (K) 126 mg, Phosphorus 79 mg

108. Curried Cauliflower

Preparation time: 5 minutes

Cooking time: 20 minutes

Servings: 4

INGREDIENTS

- 1 teaspoon turmeric
- 1 diced onion
- 1 tablespoon chopped fresh cilantro
- 1 teaspoon cumin
- ½ diced chili
- ½ cup water
- 1 minced garlic clove
- 1 tablespoon coconut oil
- 1 teaspoon garam masala
- 2 cups cauliflower florets

DIRECTIONS

1. Add the oil to a skillet on medium heat.
2. Sauté the onion and garlic for 5 minutes until soft.
3. Add in the cumin, turmeric and garam masala and stir to release the aromas.
4. Now add the chili to the pan along with the cauliflower.
5. Stir to coat.
6. Pour in the water and reduce the heat to a simmer for 15 minutes.
7. Garnish with cilantro to serve.

NUTRITION: Calories 108, Protein 2 g, Carbs 11 g, Fat 7 g, Sodium (Na) 35 mg, Potassium (K) 328 mg, Phosphorus 39 mg

109. Elegant Veggie Tortillas

Preparation Time: 30 minutes

Cooking Time: 15 minutes

Servings: 12

INGREDIENTS

- 1½ cups of chopped broccoli florets
- 1½ cups of chopped cauliflower florets
- 1 tablespoon of water
- 2 teaspoon of canola oil
- 1½ cups of chopped onion
- 1 minced garlic clove
- 2 tablespoons of finely chopped fresh parsley
- 1 cup of low-cholesterol liquid egg substitute
- Freshly ground black pepper, to taste
- 4 (6-ounce) warmed corn tortillas

DIRECTIONS

1. In a microwave bowl, place broccoli, cauliflower and water and microwave, covered for about 3-5 minutes.
2. Remove from microwave and drain any liquid.
3. Heat oil on medium heat.
4. Add onion and sauté for about 4-5 minutes.
5. Add garlic and then sauté it for about 1 minute.
6. Stir in broccoli, cauliflower, parsley, egg substitute and black pepper.
7. Reduce the heat and it to simmer for about 10 minutes.
8. Remove from heat and keep aside to cool slightly.
9. Place broccoli mixture over ¼ of each tortilla.
10. Fold the outside edges inward and roll up like a burrito.
11. Secure each tortilla with toothpicks to secure the filling.
12. Cut each tortilla in half and serve.

NUTRITION: Per Serving, Calories: 217-Fat: 3.3g - Carbs: 41g - Protein: 8.1g - Fiber: 6.3g - Potassium: 289mg - Sodium: 87mg

110. Simple Broccoli Stir-Fry

Preparation Time: 40 minutes

Cooking Time: 15 minutes

Servings: 4

INGREDIENTS

- 1 tablespoon of olive oil
- 1 minced garlic clove
- 2 cups of broccoli florets
- 2 tablespoons of water

DIRECTIONS

1. Heat oil on medium heat.
2. Add garlic and then sauté for about 1 minute.
3. Add the broccoli and stir fry for about 2 minutes.
4. Stir in water and stir fry for about 4-5 minutes.
5. Serve warm.

NUTRITION: Per Serving, Calories: 47-Fat: 3.6g - Carbs: 3.3g - Protein: 1.3g - Fiber: 1.2g - Potassium: 147mg - Sodium: 15mg

Vegetarian

111. Braised Cabbage

Preparation Time: 30 minutes

Cooking Time: 15 minutes

Servings: 4

INGREDIENTS

- 1½ teaspoon of olive oil
- 2 minced garlic cloves
- 1 thinly sliced onion
- 3 cups of chopped green cabbage
- 1 cup of low-sodium vegetable broth
- Freshly ground black pepper, to taste

DIRECTIONS

1. In a large skillet, heat oil on medium-high heat.
2. Add garlic and then sauté for about 1 minute.
3. Add onion and sauté for about 4-5 minutes.
4. Add cabbage and sauté for about 3-4 minutes.
5. Stir in broth and black pepper and immediately, reduce the heat to low.
6. Cook, covered for about 20 minutes.
7. Serve warm.

NUTRITION: Per Serving, Calories: 45-Fat: 1.8g - Carbs: 6.6g - Protein: 1.1g - Fiber: 1.9g - Potassium: 136mg - Sodium: 46mg

112. Salad with Strawberries and Goat Cheese

Preparation Time: 15 Minutes

Cooking time: 0 minute

Servings: 2

INGREDIENTS

- Baby lettuce, to taste
- 1-pint strawberries
- Balsamic vinegar
- Extra virgin olive oil
- 1/4 teaspoon black pepper
- 8-ounce soft goat cheese

DIRECTIONS

1. Prepare the lettuce by washing and drying it, then cut the strawberries.
2. Cut the soft goat cheese into 8 pieces.
3. Put together the balsamic vinegar and the extra virgin olive oil in a large cup with a whisk.
4. Mix the strawberries pressing them and putting them in a bowl, add the dressing and mix, then divide the lettuce into four dishes and cut the other strawberries, arranging them on the salad.
5. Put cheese slices on top and add pepper. Serve and enjoy!

NUTRITION: Calories: 300 Protein: 13 g Sodium: 285 mg Potassium: 400 mg Phosphorus: 193 mg

113. Roasted Veggies Mediterranean Style

Preparation Time: 5 minutes

Cooking Time: 10 minutes

Servings: 2

INGREDIENTS

- ½ teaspoon freshly grated lemon zest
- 1 cup grape tomatoes
- 1 tablespoon extra-virgin olive oil
- 1 tablespoon lemon juice
- 1 teaspoon dried oregano
- 10 pitted black olives, sliced
- 12-ounce broccoli crowns, trimmed and cut into bite-sized pieces
- 2 cloves garlic, minced
- 2 teaspoons capers, rinsed

DIRECTIONS

1. Preheat oven to 350oF and grease a baking sheet with cooking spray.
2. In a large bowl toss together until thoroughly coated salt, garlic, oil, tomatoes and broccoli. Spread broccoli on prepped baking sheet and bake for 8 to 10 minutes.
3. In another large bowl mix capers, oregano, olives, lemon juice, and lemon zest. Mix in roasted vegetables and serve while still warm.

NUTRITION: Calories: 110; carbs: 16g; protein: 6g; fats: 4g; phosphorus: 138mg; potassium: 745mg; sodium: 214mg

Fruity Garden Lettuce Salad

Preparation Time: 10 minutes

Cooking Time: 0 minutes

Servings: 4

INGREDIENTS

- ¼ cup apple cider vinegar
- ¼ cup chopped almonds
- ½ avocado, thinly sliced
- ½ cup extra virgin olive oil
- ½ lemon, juiced
- 1 teaspoon ground black pepper
- 2 Granny Smith apples, thinly sliced
- 2 teaspoons grainy mustard
- 6 cups thinly sliced lettuce

DIRECTIONS

1. In a large salad bowl, toss lemon juice and apples. Mix in almonds, avocado, and lettuce.

2. Mix salt, pepper, mustard, vinegar and olive oil until salt is thoroughly dissolved.
3. Pour in the dressing all over lettuce mixture and toss well to combine. Serve and enjoy.

NUTRITION: Calories: 123; carbs: 16.5g; protein: 2g; fats: 6g; phosphorus: 56mg; potassium: 450mg; sodium: 35mg

114. Baked Dilly Pickerel

Preparation Time: 5 minutes

Cooking Time: 15 minutes

Servings: 3

INGREDIENTS

- 4 Fillets of pickerel, about 4 ounces
- For the dilly Sauce
- ½ package of whipped cream cheese
- 4 Minced garlic cloves
- ½ Diced small onion
- 3 tablespoons of fresh or dried dill
- ½ teaspoon of ground pepper

DIRECTIONS

1. Preheat your oven to a temperature of 345°F.
2. Mix the ingredients of the dilly sauce very well to make a paste.
3. Line a baking pan with a tin foil; then set the fish and spread the dilly sauce on its top
4. Cover the fish with an aluminum foil tin and bake it for about 15 minutes in the oven
5. Serve and enjoy your dinner!

NUTRITION: Calories: 295.6, Fats: 18.7g, Carbs: 11g, Fiber: 2.2g, Potassium: 140mg, Sodium: 6.8mg, Phosphorous: 58g, Protein 20.7g

115. Rice Salad

Preparation Time: 10 minutes

Cooking Time: 20 minutes

Servings: 2

INGREDIENTS

- 1 Cup of olive oil
- ½ Cup of balsamic vinegar
- 1 teaspoon of lemon juice
- ¾ teaspoons of black pepper
- 3 Minced garlic cloves
- ½ teaspoon of dried basil
- ½ teaspoon of dried oregano
- ½ Cup of fresh parsley
- 2 cups of bell peppers
- ½ Cup of chopped red onion
- 1 Cup of frozen artichoke hearts
- 1/3 Cup of fresh dill weed
- 6 Cups of cooked white rice
- 1 Pound of cooked shrimp
- ½ Cup of dried cranberries
- 8 Ounces of canned pineapple chunks
- 1 Cup of frozen green peas

DIRECTIONS

1. To make the dressing, whisk all together the oil with the vinegar, the salt, the pepper, the minced garlic, the basil, the oregano and about ¼ cup of chopped parsley; then set the mixture aside.
2. Chop the red bell peppers and the onion; then mince the dill weed
3. Cook your ingredients and quarter the artichoke hearts.
4. In a large bowl combine the rice with the shrimp, the bell peppers, the onion, the artichoke hearts, and ½ cup of minced parsley, the dill, the cranberries, the pineapple and the green peas.
5. Stir the dressing and let it chill for about 2 hours to marinate.
6. Serve and enjoy your dinner over a bed of lettuce!

NUTRITION: Calories: 165.4, Fats: 11g, Carbs: 8g, Fiber: 0.89g, Potassium: 181mg, Sodium:99mg, Phosphorous: 75g, Protein 8g

116. Baked Eggplant Tray

Preparation time: 10 minutes

Cooking Time: 20 minutes

Servings: 2

INGREDIENTS

- 3 Cups of eggplant
- 3 large omega-3 eggs
- ½ Cup of liquid non-dairy creamer
- 1 teaspoon of vinegar
- 1 Teaspoon of lemon juice
- ½ teaspoon of pepper
- ¼ teaspoon of sage
- ½ Cup of white breadcrumbs
- 1 tablespoon of margarine

DIRECTIONS

1. Preheat the oven to a temperature of about 350°F
2. Peel the eggplant and cut it into pieces
3. Place the eggplant pieces in a large pan; then cover it with water and let boil until it becomes tender
4. Drain the eggplants and mash it very well
5. Combine the beaten eggs with the non-dairy creamer, the vinegar, the lemon juice, the pepper

and the sage with the mashed eggplant; then place it into a greased baking tray
6. Mix the melted margarine with the breadcrumbs.
7. Top you tray with the breadcrumbs and bake it for about 20 minutes
8. Set the tray aside to cool for about 5 minutes
9. Serve and enjoy your dinner!

NUTRITION: Calories: 126, Fats: 8g, Carbs: 4.7g, Fiber: 1.6g, Potassium: 224mg, Sodium: 143mg, Phosphorous: 115g, Protein 7.3g

117. Raw Vegetables. Chopped Salad

Preparation Time: 15 minutes

Cooking Time: 0 minute

Servings: 4

INGREDIENTS

- Chopped raw veggie salad
- 1 orange pepper (minced) (about 1 cup)
- 1 yellow pepper (small cut) (about 1 cup)
- 5-8 radishes (halve and cut into thin slices) (about 3/4 cup)
- small head of broccoli (minced) (about 2 cups)
- 1 seedless cucumber (small cut) (about 2 cups)
- 1 cup of halved red seedless grapes
- 2-3 tablespoons chopped fresh dill
- 1/4 cup chopped fresh parsley
- 1/4 cup of raw peeled sunflower seeds
- 1/8 cup raw hemp hearts (peeled hemp seeds)
- Oil-free dressing
- garlic clove (chopped)
- tablespoons of red wine vinegar
- 1 tablespoon of apple cider vinegar
- Juice of 1 lemon
- 1 tablespoon Dijonsenf
- 1 tablespoon pure maple syrup
- 1/2 teaspoon salt (or to taste)
- 1/8 teaspoon pepper (or to taste)

DIRECTIONS

1. Whisk the ingredients - Chopped raw veggie salad, 1 orange pepper, yellow pepper, radishes, small head of broccoli, seedless cucumber, halved red seedless grapes, chopped fresh dill, chopped fresh parsley, raw peeled sunflower seeds, raw hemp hearts, garlic clove, red wine vinegar, apple cider vinegar, lemon, Dijonsenf, pure maple syrup, salt, pepper. For dressing in a small bowl and set aside.
2. Mix all the salad ingredients in a large bowl.
3. Pour the dressing over and wrap well.
4. Cover and then refrigerate it for an hour or two and toss the salad once or twice during this time to coat evenly. Enjoy!

NUTRITION: Calories: 111 Total Fat: 2g Saturated Fat: 1g Cholesterol: 10mg Sodium: 58mg Carbohydrates: 19g Sugar: 18 g Calcium: 15%

118. Mediterranean Veggie Pita Sandwich

Preparation Time: 4hours: 30mins

Cooking Time: 30 minutes

Servings: 2

INGREDIENTS

- 1/4 cup chopped carrots
- A handful of baby spinach
- 1/4 cup chickpeas
- 1 teaspoon of crumbled feta cheese
- 2 teaspoons of fine chopped sun-dried tomatoes
- 2 teaspoons of chopped kalamata olives
- Season with salt and pepper

DIRECTIONS

1. The chopped carrots, baby spinach, chickpeas, crumbled feta cheese, chopped sun-dried tomatoes, chopped kalamata olives, salt and pepper. Spread the bath in every pita pant. Sort the rest of the ingredients between the boxes. Eat immediately or pack in a container for lunch. Cool the device if you prepare it for more than 4 hours before eating.

NUTRITION: Calories 287.6 Sodium 716.0 mg Potassium 263.6 mg Total Carbohydrate 45.7 g Dietary Fiber 6.8 g

119. Classic asparagus

Preparation Time: 20 minutes

Cooking Time: 20 minutes

Servings: 4

INGREDIENTS

- 2 kg of white asparagus
- 12 pieces medium potatoes
- 4 eggs
- 1 first-class salt
- 1 premium sugar
- 1 tablespoon butter
- For the sauce:
- 200 g butter
- 2 egg yolks
- 4 tablespoons white wine
- 1 tablespoon lemon juice
- 1 first-class salt
- 1 premium white pepper

DIRECTIONS

1. Cook the peeled asparagus in plenty of hot water (seasoned with salt, sugar, and butter) for 15 - 20 minutes.
2. Peel the potatoes and cook as usual or cool with the air freezer. The eggs are cooked hard.
3. for the sauce: Dissolve the butter in a hot freezer and allow cooling slightly.
4. Grease the egg yolks with lemon juice and white wine in a warm water bath until the mass is thick.
5. Then the cooled and melted butter is slowed down slowly. Now the sauce is seasoned with salt and pepper.
6. Tips on the recipe
7. Distribute the asparagus in 4 portions and arrange with potatoes and the halved eggs on 4 plates.

NUTRITION: Calories 20 % daily value Total fat 0.1 g 0% Saturated fat 0 g 0% Total carbohydrate 3.9 g 1% Dietary fiber 2.1 g 8% Sugar 1.9 g Protein 2.2 g 4%

120. Vegetarian Pasticcio

Preparation Time: 10 minutes

Cooking Time: 30 minutes

Servings: 4

INGREDIENTS

- 7 eggs
- 7 slices of sourdough bread
- 1-ounce shredded sharp cheddar cheese
- 1 piece of onion
- 1 cup of raw mushrooms
- 1 cup red bell peppers
- 15 fresh spinach leaves
- ½ teaspoon black pepper
- ¼ glass vinegar§
- 3 portions of half and half cream
- Worcestershire sauce (1 teaspoon)
- Hot sauce (1 teaspoon)
- Unsalted margarine (1 teaspoon)

DIRECTIONS

1. Cut onion, pepper and mushrooms into small dices.
2. Chop bread into small dices and place on a baking sheet. Bake in the oven at 225°F (or 100°C) for 15 minutes, turning the cubes every 15 minutes and then still cook them for other 15 minutes.
3. Put onion, pepper and mushrooms mix in a skillet pre-greased with olive oil.
4. Grease a dish and put in it both bread dices and the vegetable mixture, then put the spinach leaves on top. Arrange for a second layer of the same mixture.
5. Put together the half and half cream with eggs, vinegar, Worcestershire sauce, hot sauce and black pepper. Pour this mix over the bread. Put the covered dish in the fridge for one hour. When out of the fridge, put the dish aside for at least 20 minutes.
6. Preheat oven at 330 °F. Bake for 50 minutes without the covering and when you take it out of the oven, sprinkle the cheddar cheese over the top. Cook for 10 minutes and cut into 10 slices and serve it hot.

NUTRITION: 210 calories10 g protein15 g carbohydrates10 g fat165 mg cholesterol215 mg sodium345 mg potassium205 mg phosphorus150 mg calcium2.0 fiber

121. Cauliflower and Asparagus Tortilla

Preparation Time: 10 minutes

Cooking Time: 30 minutes

Servings: 4

INGREDIENTS

- Asparagus – 2 cups
- Cauliflower – 2 cups
- Olive oil – 2 teaspoons
- Onion – 1½ cups
- Garlic – 1 clove
- Liquid egg substitute (low-cholesterol) – 1 cup
- Fresh parsley (finely chopped) – 2 tablespoons
- Salt – ¼ teaspoon
- Pepper (freshly ground) – ½ teaspoon
- Dried thyme leaves (crushed) – ¼ teaspoon
- Ground nutmeg – ¼ teaspoon

DIRECTIONS

1. Start by chopping the asparagus and cauliflower into 1-inch pieces. Take the onion and chop it finely. Also, mince the garlic clove.
2. Take a microwave-safe bowl and place the chopped cauliflower and asparagus pieces into it. Add in 1 tablespoon of water and cover the dish.
3. After that, drain any excess water and set aside.
4. Microwave them for about 4-5 minutes. Make sure the veggies are slightly tender.
5. Place a saucepan over a high flame and pour the oil into it. Once heated, toss in the finely chopped onions.
6. Sauté the onions for about 6-7 minutes. Add in the minced garlic and sauté for 1 more minute.
7. Toss in the cauliflower, asparagus, egg substitute, salt, thyme, parsley, and nutmeg. Arrange them well over the egg substitute base.

8. Cover the saucepan, and cook for about 15 minutes in low heat.
9. Use a butter knife to loosen the edges of the prepared tortilla.
10. Take a microwave-safe serving platter and heat it for about 30-40 seconds.
11. Invert the tortilla onto the heated serving platter. Serve hot!

NUTRITION: Protein – 9 g Fat – 3 g Carbohydrates – 9 g Sodium – 248 mg Cholesterol – 0 mg Potassium – 472 mg Calcium – 68 mg Phosphorus – 97 mg Fiber – 3.88 g

SNACKS AND SIDE

122. Fluffy Mock Pancakes

Preparation Time: 5 minutes

Cooking Time: 10 minutes

Servings: 2

INGREDIENTS

- 1 egg
- 1 cup ricotta cheese
- 1 teaspoon cinnamon
- 2 tablespoons honey, add more if needed

DIRECTIONS

1. Using a blender, put together egg, honey, cinnamon, and ricotta cheese. Process until all ingredients are well combined.
2. Pour an equal amount of the blended mixture into the pan. Cook each pancake for 4 minutes on both sides. Serve.

NUTRITION: Calories: 188.1 kcal Total Fat: 14.5 g Saturated Fat: 4.5 g Cholesterol: 139.5 mg Sodium: 175.5 mg Total Carbs: 5.5 g Fiber: 2.8 g Sugar: 0.9 g Protein: 8.5 g

123. Mixes of Snack

Preparation Time: 10 minutes

Cooking Time: 1 hours and 15 minutes

Servings: 4

INGREDIENTS

- 6 cup margarine
- 2 tablespoon Worcestershire sauce
- 1 ½ tablespoon spice salt
- ¾ cup garlic powder
- ½ teaspoon onion powder
- 3 cups Crispi
- 3 cups Cheerios
- 3 cups corn flakes
- 1 cup KIXE
- 1 cup pretzels
- 1 cup broken bagel chips into 1-inch pieces

DIRECTIONS

1. Preheat the oven to 250F (120C)
2. Melt the margarine in a pan. Stir in the seasoning. Gradually add the ingredients remaining by mixing so that the coating is uniform.
3. Cook 1 hour, stirring every 15 minutes. Spread on paper towels to let cool. Store in a tightly-closed container.

NUTRITION: Calories: 200 kcal Total Fat: 9 g Saturated Fat: 3.5 g Cholesterol: 0 mg Sodium: 3.5 mg Total Carbs: 27 g Fiber: 2 g Sugar: 0 g Protein: 3 g

124. Cranberry Dip with Fresh Fruit

Preparation time: 10 minutes

Cooking time: 0 minutes

Servings: 8

INGREDIENTS

- 8-ounce sour cream
- 1/2 cup whole berry cranberry sauce
- 1/4 teaspoon nutmeg
- 1/4 teaspoon ground ginger
- 4 cups fresh pineapple, peeled, cubed
- 4 medium apples, peeled, cored and cubed
- 4 medium pears, peeled, cored and cubed
- 1 teaspoon lemon juice

DIRECTIONS

1. Start by adding cranberry sauce, sour cream, ginger, and nutmeg to a food processor.
2. Blend the mixture until its smooth then transfer it to a bowl.
3. Toss the pineapple, with pears, apples, and lemon juice in a salad bowl.
4. Thread the fruits onto mini skewers.
5. Serve them with the sauce.

NUTRITION: Calories 70. Protein 0 g. Carbohydrates 13 g. Fat 2 g. Cholesterol 4 mg. Sodium 8 mg. Potassium 101 mg. Phosphorus 15 mg. Calcium 17 mg. Fiber 1.5 g.

125. Cucumbers with Sour Cream

Preparation time: 10 minutes

Cooking time: 0 minutes

Servings: 4

INGREDIENTS

- 2 medium cucumbers, peeled and sliced thinly
- 1/2 medium sweet onion, sliced
- 1/4 cup white wine vinegar
- 1 tablespoon canola oil
- 1/8 teaspoon black pepper
- 1/2 cup reduced-fat sour cream

DIRECTIONS

1. Toss in cucumber, onion, and all other ingredients in a medium-size bowl.
2. Mix well and refrigerate for 2 hours.
3. Toss again and serve to enjoy.

NUTRITION: Calories 64. Protein 1 g. Carbohydrates 4 g. Fat 5 g. Cholesterol 3 mg. Sodium 72 mg. Potassium 113 mg. Phosphorus 24 mg. Calcium 21 mg. Fiber 0.8 g.

126. Sweet Savory Meatballs

Preparation time: 10 minutes

Cooking time: 20 minutes

Servings: 12

INGREDIENTS

- 1-pound ground turkey
- 1 large egg
- 1/4 cup bread crumbs
- 2 tablespoon onion, finely chopped
- 1 teaspoon garlic powder
- 1/2 teaspoon black pepper
- 1/4 cup canola oil
- 6-ounce grape jelly
- 1/4 cup chili sauce

DIRECTIONS

1. Place all ingredients except chili sauce and jelly in a large mixing bowl.
2. Mix well until evenly mixed then make small balls out of this mixture.
3. It will make about 48 meatballs. Spread them out on a greased pan on a stovetop.
4. Cook them over medium heat until brown on all the sides.
5. Mix chili sauce with jelly in a microwave-safe bowl and heat it for 2 minutes in the microwave.
6. Pour this chili sauce mixture onto the meatballs in the pan.
7. Transfer the meatballs in the pan to the preheated oven.
8. Bake the meatballs for 20 minutes in an oven at 375 degrees F.
9. Serve fresh and warm.

NUTRITION: Calories 127. Protein 9 g. Carbohydrates 14 g. Fat 4 g. Cholesterol 41 mg. Sodium 129 mg. Potassium 148 mg. Phosphorus 89 mg. Calcium 15 mg. Fiber 0.2 g.

127. Spicy Corn Bread

Preparation time: 10 minutes

Cooking time: 30 minutes

Servings: 8

INGREDIENTS

- 1 cup all-purpose white flour
- 1 cup plain cornmeal
- 1 tablespoon sugar
- 2 teaspoon baking powder
- 1 teaspoon chili powder
- 1/4 teaspoon black pepper
- 1 cup rice milk, unenriched
- 1 egg
- 1 egg white
- 2 tablespoon canola oil
- 1/2 cup scallions, finely chopped
- 1/4 cup carrots, finely grated
- 1 garlic clove, minced

DIRECTIONS

1. Preheat your oven to 400 degrees F.
2. Now start by mixing the flour with baking powder, sugar, cornmeal, pepper and chili powder in a mixing bowl.
3. Stir in oil, milk, egg white, and egg.
4. Mix well until it's smooth then stir in carrots, garlic, and scallions.
5. Stir well then spread the batter in an 8-inch baking pan greased with cooking spray.
6. Bake for 30 minutes until golden brown.
7. Slice and serve fresh.

NUTRITION: Calories 188. Protein 5 g. Carbohydrates 31 g. Fat 5 g. Cholesterol 26 mg. Sodium 155 mg. Potassium 100 mg. Phosphorus 81 mg. Calcium 84 mg. Fiber 2 g.

128. Sweet and Spicy Tortilla Chips

Preparation time: 10 minutes

Cooking time: 8 minutes

Servings: 6

INGREDIENTS

- 1/4 cup butter
- 1 teaspoon brown sugar
- 1/2 teaspoon ground chili powder
- 1/2 teaspoon garlic powder
- 1/2 teaspoon ground cumin
- 1/4 teaspoon ground cayenne pepper
- 6 flour tortillas, 6" size

DIRECTIONS

1. Preheat oven to 425 degrees F.
2. Grease a baking sheet with cooking spray.
3. Add all spices, brown sugar, and melted butter to a small bowl.
4. Mix well and set this mixture aside.
5. Slice the tortillas into 8 wedges and brush them with the sugar mixture.
6. Spread them on the baking sheet and bake them for 8 minutes.
7. Serve fresh.

NUTRITION: Calories 115. Protein 2 g. Carbohydrates 11 g. Fat 7 g. Cholesterol 15 mg. Sodium 156 mg. Potassium 42 mg. Phosphorus 44 mg. Calcium 31 mg. Fiber 0.6 g.

129. Addictive Pretzels

Preparation time: 10 minutes

Cooking time: 1 hour

Servings: 6

INGREDIENTS

- 32-ounce bag unsalted pretzels
- 1 cup canola oil
- 2 tablespoon seasoning mix
- 3 teaspoon garlic powder
- 3 teaspoon dried dill weed

DIRECTIONS

1. Preheat oven to 175 degrees F.
2. Place the pretzels on a cooking sheet and break them into pieces.
3. Mix garlic powder and dill in a bowl and reserve half of the mixture.
4. Mix the remaining half with seasoning mix and ¾ cup of canola oil.
5. Pour this oil over the pretzels and brush them liberally
6. Bake the pieces for 1 hour then flip them to bake for another 15 minutes.
7. Allow them to cool then sprinkle the remaining dill mixture and drizzle more oil on top.
8. Serve fresh and warm.

NUTRITION: Calories 184. Protein 2 g. Carbohydrates 22 g. Fat 8 g. Cholesterol 0 mg. Sodium 60 mg. Potassium 43 mg. Phosphorus 28 mg. Calcium 2 mg. Fiber 1.0 g.

130. Shrimp Spread with Crackers

Preparation time: 10 minutes

Cooking time: 0 minutes

Servings: 6

INGREDIENTS

- 1/4 cup light cream cheese
- 2 1/2-ounce cooked, shelled shrimp, minced
- 1 tablespoon no-salt-added ketchup
- 1/4 teaspoon hot sauce
- 1 teaspoon Worcestershire sauce
- 1/2 teaspoon herb seasoning blend
- 24 matzo cracker miniatures
- 1 tablespoon parsley

DIRECTIONS

1. Start by tossing the minced shrimp with cream cheese in a bowl.
2. Stir in Worcestershire sauce, hot sauce, herb seasoning, and ketchup.
3. Mix well and garnish with minced parsley.
4. Serve the spread with the crackers.

NUTRITION: Calories 57. Protein 3 g. Carbohydrates 7 g. Fat 1 g. Cholesterol 21 mg. Sodium 69 mg. Potassium 54 mg. Phosphorus 30 mg. Calcium 15 mg. Fiber 0.2 g.

131. Buffalo Chicken Dip

Preparation time: 10 minutes

Cooking time: 3 hours

Servings: 4

INGREDIENTS

- 4-ounce cream cheese
- 1/2 cup bottled roasted red peppers
- 1 cup reduced-fat sour cream
- 4 teaspoon hot pepper sauce
- 2 cups cooked, shredded chicken

DIRECTIONS

1. Blend half cup of drained red peppers in a food processor until smooth.
2. Now, thoroughly mix cream cheese, and sour cream with the pureed peppers in a bowl.
3. Stir in shredded chicken and hot sauce then transfer the mixture to a slow cooker.
4. Cook for 3 hours on low heat.
5. Serve warm with celery, carrots, cauliflower, and cucumber.

NUTRITION: Calories 73. Protein 5 g. Carbohydrates 2 g. Fat 5 g. Cholesterol 25 mg. Sodium 66 mg. Potassium 81 mg. Phosphorus 47 mg. Calcium 31 mg. Fiber 0 g.

132. Chicken Pepper Bacon Wraps

Preparation time: 10 minutes

Cooking time: 15 minutes

Servings: 4

INGREDIENTS

- 1 medium onion, chopped
- 12 strips bacon, halved
- 12 fresh jalapenos peppers
- 12 fresh banana peppers
- 2 pounds boneless, skinless chicken breast

DIRECTIONS

1. How to prepare:
2. Grease a grill rack with cooking spray and preheat the grill on low heat.
3. Slice the peppers in half lengthwise then remove their seeds.
4. Dice the chicken into small pieces and divide them into each pepper.

5. Now spread the chopped onion over the chicken in the peppers.
6. Wrap the bacon strips around the stuffed peppers.
7. Place these wrapped peppers in the grill and cook them for 15 minutes.
8. Serve fresh and warm.

NUTRITION: Calories 71. Protein 10 g. Carbohydrates 1 g. Fat 3 g. Cholesterol 26 mg. Sodium 96 mg. Potassium 147 mg. Phosphorus 84 mg. Calcium 9 mg. Fiber 0.8 g.

133. Garlic Oyster Crackers

Preparation time: 10 minutes

Cooking time: 45 minutes

Servings: 4

INGREDIENTS

- 1/2 cup butter-flavored popcorn oil
- 1 tablespoon garlic powder
- 7 cups oyster crackers
- 2 teaspoon dried dill weed

DIRECTIONS

1. How to prepare:
2. Preheat oven to 250 degrees F.
3. Mix garlic powder with oil in a large bowl.
4. Toss in crackers and mix well to coat evenly.
5. Sprinkle the dill weed over the crackers and toss well again.
6. Spread the crackers on the baking sheet and bake them for 45 minutes.
7. Toss them every 15 minutes.
8. Serve fresh.

NUTRITION: Calories 118. Protein 2 g. Carbohydrates 12 g. Fat 7 g. Cholesterol 0 mg. Sodium 166 mg. Potassium 21 mg. Phosphorus 15 mg. Calcium 4 mg. Fiber 3 g.

134. Lime Cilantro Rice

Preparation Time: 5 minutes

Cooking Time: 20 minutes

Servings: 2

INGREDIENTS

- White rice – .75 cup
- Water – 1.5 cups
- Olive oil – 1.5 tablespoons
- Bay leaf, ground - .25 teaspoon
- Lime juice – 1 tablespoon
- Lemon juice – 1 tablespoon
- Lime zest - .25 teaspoon
- Cilantro, chopped - .25 cup

DIRECTIONS

1. Place the white rice and water in a medium-sized saucepan and bring it to a boil over medium heat. Simmer and cover the pot with a lid, allowing it to cook until all water has been absorbed about eighteen to twenty minutes.
2. Stir in the ground bay leaf, olive oil, lime juice, lemon juice, lime zest, and cilantro after cooking. You want to do this with a fork, preferably, as this will fluff the rice rather than causing it to compact. Serve while warm.

NUTRITION: Calories in Individual Servings: 363 Protein Grams: 5 Phosphorus Milligrams: 74 Potassium Milligrams: 86 Sodium Milligrams: 5 Fat Grams: 10 Total Carbohydrates Grams: 60 Net Carbohydrates Grams: 58

135. Spanish Rice

Preparation Time: 5 minutes

Cooking Time: 20 minutes

Servings: 2

INGREDIENTS

- White rice – .75 cup
- Chicken broth, low sodium– 1.5 cups
- Onion dehydrated flakes – 2 tablespoons
- Garlic, minced – 2 cloves
- Lemon juice – 1 tablespoon
- Cumin, ground - .25 teaspoon
- Chili powder - .5 teaspoon
- Oregano, dried - .5 teaspoon
- Black pepper, ground - .25 teaspoon
- Cilantro, chopped – 3 tablespoons

DIRECTIONS

1. Place the rice, chicken broth, onion flakes, and minced garlic in a medium-sized saucepan. Bring the chicken broth and the rice to a boil over medium heat, and then reduce the heat to a light simmer, cover it with a lid, and allow it to cook until the liquid has all been absorbed about eighteen to twenty minutes.
2. Use a fork to fluff the rice mix in the lemon juice, cumin, chili powder, oregano, black pepper, and cilantro. Once combined, serve the rice while still warm.

NUTRITION: Calories in Individual Servings: 303 Protein Grams: 6 Phosphorus Milligrams: 104 Potassium Milligrams: 197 Sodium Milligrams: 57 Fat Grams: 1 Total Carbohydrates Grams: 65 Net Carbohydrates Grams: 63

136. Parmesan Quinoa with Peas

Preparation Time: 5 minutes

Cooking Time: 20 minutes

Servings: 2

INGREDIENTS

- Quinoa – .75 cup
- Water – 1.5 cups
- Green peas, thawed if frozen - .75 cup
- Black pepper, ground - .25 teaspoon
- Olive oil – 1.5 tablespoons
- Parmesan cheese, grated – 3 tablespoons

DIRECTIONS

1. Place the uncooked quinoa in a fine metal sieve and rinse it well with water until there is no debris running off.
2. Place the quinoa and water in a metal saucepan and bring it to a boil over medium heat. Once it attains a boil, reduce it to a light simmer, cover the pot with a lid, and allow cooking until the water has all been absorbed. This should take fifteen to twenty minutes.
3. Allow the quinoa to sit with the lid on for five minutes after turning off the heat. Once it has set, use a fork to fluff the quinoa and stir in the green peas, olive oil, and quinoa. Close the lid once again, allowing it to sit for five additional minutes to warm the peas and melt the cheese. Enjoy the quinoa while warm.

NUTRITION: Calories in Individual Servings: 386 Protein Grams: 13 Phosphorus Milligrams: 378 Potassium Milligrams: 465 Sodium Milligrams: 144 Fat Grams: 16 Total Carbohydrates Grams: 47 Net Carbohydrates Grams: 41

137. Mushroom Orzo

Preparation Time: 5 minutes

Cooking Time: 20 minutes

Servings: 2

INGREDIENTS

- Orzo - .75 cup
- Chicken broth, low-sodium – 1.25 cup
- Mushrooms, diced – 4 ounces
- Garlic, minced – 3 cloves
- Onion flakes, dehydrated – 1 tablespoon
- Olive oil – 1 tablespoon
- Sage, ground - .25 teaspoon

DIRECTIONS

1. Place the diced mushrooms, olive oil, and garlic in a medium-sized metal saucepan and allow them to sauté over medium heat for five minutes. Add in the sage, onion flakes, orzo, and low-sodium chicken broth. Bring the mixture to a boil.
2. Reduce the heat of the skillet to a light simmer, cover the pot with a lid, and allow it to cook until all of the liquid has been absorbed about nine minutes. Fluff the orzo with a fork before serving.

NUTRITION: Calories in Individual Servings: 337 Protein Grams: 18 Phosphorus Milligrams: 63 Potassium Milligrams: 430 Sodium Milligrams: 43 Fat Grams: 8 Total Carbohydrates Grams: 99 Net Carbohydrates Grams: 95

138. Carrot and Pineapple Slaw

Preparation Time: 5 minutes

Cooking Time: 0 minute

Servings: 2

INGREDIENTS

- Carrot matchsticks – 5 ounces
- Pineapple chunks, canned, liquid drained - .5 cup
- Grapes, sliced in half - .5 cup
- Pecan pieces - .25 cup
- Mayonnaise, low-sodium - .33 cup
- Lemon juice – 1 tablespoon

DIRECTIONS

1. In a bowl, toss together the carrot matchsticks, drained pineapple chunks, sliced grapes, and pecan pieces. Stir in the low-sodium mayonnaise and lemon juice.
2. Cover the bowl with plastic wrap or a lid and then allow it to chill and marinate for at least an hour before serving. You can make this slaw up to a day in advance.

NUTRITION: Calories in Individual Servings: 264 Protein Grams: 2 Phosphorus Milligrams: 74 Potassium Milligrams: 423 Sodium Milligrams: 91 Fat Grams: 17 Total Carbohydrates Grams: 29 Net Carbohydrates Grams: 25

139. Sesame Cucumber Salad

Preparation Time: 5 minutes

Cooking Time: 0 minute

Servings: 2

INGREDIENTS

- Cucumbers, thinly sliced – 1
- Sesame seeds - .5 teaspoon
- Rice wine vinegar – 1 tablespoon
- Sugar - .5 tablespoon
- Sesame seed oil – 1.5 tablespoons
- Red pepper flakes - .25 teaspoon

DIRECTIONS

1. You want the cucumbers sliced as thinly as you can get them. While you can certainly do this with a knife, it is quicker and easier if you use a mandolin.
2. In a medium to a small bowl, whisk together the sesame seeds, rice wine vinegar, sugar, sesame seed oil, and red pepper flakes. Once well combined, add in the cucumbers and toss the vegetables in the vinaigrette. Serve immediately.

NUTRITION: Calories in Individual Servings: 92 Protein Grams: 1 Phosphorus Milligrams: 46 Potassium Milligrams: 250 Sodium Milligrams: 117 Fat Grams: 5

140. Creamy Jalapeno Corn

Preparation Time: 5 minutes

Cooking Time: 15 minutes

Servings: 2

INGREDIENTS

- Corn kernels, fresh – 1 cup
- Red bell pepper, diced - .25 cup
- Jalapeno, seeded and diced – 1
- Cream cheese – 1.5 ounces
- Olive oil – 1 tablespoon
- Black pepper, ground - .25 teaspoon
- Cheddar cheese, low-sodium - .25 cup

DIRECTIONS

1. Preheat your oven to a Fahrenheit temperature of three-hundred and fifty degrees.
2. In a medium saucepan, sauté the bell pepper and jalapeno in the olive oil until softened, about four minutes. Add in the cream cheese and continue to stir until it melts and combines with the vegetables.
3. Add in the corn, black pepper, and half of the cheese. After the mixture is combined, sprinkle the remaining cheese over the top and place the saucepan in the oven to cook until it is hot and bubbling about fifteen minutes.

NUTRITION: Calories in Individual Servings: 284 Protein Grams: 7 Phosphorus Milligrams: 200 Potassium Milligrams: 293 Sodium Milligrams: 82 Fat Grams: 19 Total Carbohydrates Grams: 20 Net Carbohydrates Grams: 18

141. Crispy Parmesan Cauliflower

Preparation Time: 5 minutes

Cooking Time: 30 minutes

Servings: 2

INGREDIENTS

- Cauliflower florets – 2 cups
- Black pepper, ground - .125 teaspoon
- Garlic, minced – 2 cloves
- Parmesan cheese, grated – 2 tablespoons
- Bread crumbs, plain - .25 cup
- Olive oil – 1 tablespoon

DIRECTIONS

1. Preheat your oven to a Fahrenheit temperature of four-hundred degrees and line a baking sheet with kitchen parchment.
2. In one small bowl, combine the olive oil and the garlic. In another, combine the Parmesan cheese, bread crumbs, and black pepper.
3. Dip the cauliflower piece-by-piece first into the olive oil mixture, and then into the bread crumb mixture. After you coat each piece, set it on the kitchen parchment-lined sheet.
4. Place the cauliflower sheet in the middle of the oven and roast the cauliflower until it reaches golden brown perfection, about thirty minutes. Serve it immediately, while it is still warm and crispy.

NUTRITION: Calories in Individual Servings: 106 Protein Grams: 5 Phosphorus Milligrams: 166 Potassium Milligrams: 369 Sodium Milligrams: 222 Fat Grams: 9 Total Carbohydrates Grams: 16 Net Carbohydrates Grams: 14

142. Cucumber Dill Salad with Greek Yogurt Dressing

Preparation Time: 5 minutes

Cooking Time: 0 minute

Servings: 2

INGREDIENTS

- Cucumbers, cut thinly – 2
- Red onion, small, thinly sliced - .5
- Greek yogurt, plain – 3 tablespoons
- Honey – 2 teaspoons
- White vinegar – 4 teaspoons
- Black pepper, ground - .125 teaspoon
- Garlic powder - .125 teaspoon
- Dill, fresh, chopped – 1.5 tablespoons

DIRECTIONS

1. Use either a knife or a mandolin to cut the cucumbers into thin and even slices, about .25 of an inch thick.
2. In a medium bowl, whisk together the fresh dill, garlic powder, black pepper, white vinegar, honey, and Greek yogurt.
3. Into the bowl with the prepared Greek yogurt dressing, add the cucumbers and red onion, and toss them together until fully coated. Cover the

bowl with a lid or plastic wrap and allow it to chill in the fridge for at least an hour before enjoying. You can make this salad up to a day in advance.

NUTRITION: Calories in Individual Servings: 106 Protein Grams: 5 Phosphorus Milligrams: 166 Potassium Milligrams: 369 Sodium Milligrams: 222 Fat Grams: 9 Total Carbohydrates Grams: 16 Net Carbohydrates Grams: 14

143. Zesty Green Beans with Almonds

Preparation Time: 5 minutes

Cooking Time: 10 minutes

Servings: 2

INGREDIENTS

- Green beans, trimmed - .5 pound
- Olive oil – 1 tablespoon
- Shallot, diced – 1
- Garlic, minced – 2 cloves
- Almonds, sliced – 2 tablespoons
- Lemon zest - .25 teaspoon
- Lemon juice – 1 teaspoon
- Black pepper, ground - .125 teaspoon

DIRECTIONS

1. In a large skillet, sauté the shallot and garlic in the olive oil over medium heat until soft, about three minutes. Add in the green beans and black pepper and continue to cook the green beans until they are tender about seven minutes.
2. Once the green beans are ready, stir in the lemon juice and lemon zest, and then top the skillet off with the sliced almonds.

NUTRITION: Calories in Individual Servings: 143 Protein Grams: 3 Phosphorus Milligrams: 84 Potassium Milligrams: 322 Sodium Milligrams: 8 Fat Grams: 10 Total Carbohydrates Grams: 11 Net Carbohydrates Grams: 8

144. Dill Orzo

Preparation Time: 10 minutes

Cooking time: 9 minutes

Servings: 2

INGREDIENTS

- ½ cup orzo
- 1 ½ cup chicken stock
- ¼ cup fresh dill, chopped
- 1 teaspoon butter, softened

DIRECTIONS

1. Place orzo in the pan. Add chicken stock. Boil orzo for 9 minutes. Meanwhile, churn together butter with fresh dill. Combine together cooked orzo with dill butter.

NUTRITION: calories 198, fat 3.4, fiber 2.3, carbs 35.7, protein 7

145. Quinoa Tabbouleh

Preparation Time: 15 minutes

Cooking time: 10 minutes

Servings: 8

INGREDIENTS

- 1 cup quinoa
- 4 teaspoons lemon juice
- ¼ teaspoon garlic clove, diced
- 5 tablespoons sesame oil
- 2 cucumbers, chopped
- 1/3 teaspoon ground black pepper
- 1/3 cup tomatoes, chopped
- ½ ounce scallions, chopped
- ¼ teaspoon fresh mint, chopped

DIRECTIONS

1. Pour water in the pan. Add quinoa and boil it for 10 minutes. Then close the lid and let it rest for 5 minutes more. Meanwhile, in the mixing bowl mix up together lemon juice, diced garlic, sesame oil, cucumbers, ground black pepper, tomatoes, scallions, and fresh mint.
2. Then add cooked quinoa and carefully mix the side dish with the help of the spoon.
3. Store tabbouleh up to 2 days in the fridge.

NUTRITION: calories 168, fat 9.9, fiber 2, carbs 16.9, protein 3.6

146. Papaya Mint Water

Preparation time: 5 minutes

Cooking time: 0 minutes

Servings: 10

INGREDIENTS:

- 1 cup fresh papaya, peeled, seeded, and diced
- 2 tablespoons chopped fresh mint leaves
- 10 cups distilled or filtered water

DIRECTION:

1. Place the papaya and mint in a large pitcher. Pour in the water.
2. Stir, and place the pitcher in the refrigerator to infuse, overnight if possible.
3. Serve cold.

NUTRITION: Calories: 2; Total fat: 0g; Cholesterol: 0g; Sodium: 0g; Phosphorus: 0mg; Potassium: 4mg;

147. Carrot Peach Water

Preparation time: 10 minutes

Cooking time: 0 minutes

Servings: 10

INGREDIENTS:

- 2 peaches, peeled, pitted, and chopped
- 1 large carrot, peeled and grated
- 1-inch piece peeled fresh ginger, lightly crushed
- 3 fresh thyme sprigs
- 10 cups water

DIRECTION:

1. Place the peaches, carrot, ginger, and thyme in a large pitcher.
2. Pour in the water, and stir the mixture.
3. Place the pitcher in the refrigerator and leave to infuse, overnight if possible.
4. Serve cold.

NUTRITION: Calories: 3; Total fat: 0g; Sodium: 0g; Phosphorus: 0mg; Potassium: 4mg;

148. Corn Bread

Preparation time: 10 minutes

Cooking time: 20 minutes

Servings: 10

INGREDIENTS:

- Cooking spray for greasing the baking dish
- Yellow cornmeal – 1 ¼ cups
- All-purpose flour – ¾ cup
- Baking soda substitute – 1 tablespoon
- Granulated sugar – ½ cup
- Eggs – 2
- Unsweetened, unfortified rice milk – 1 cup
- Olive oil – 2 Tablespoons.

DIRECTION:

1. Preheat the oven to 425F.
2. Lightly spray an 8-by-8-inch baking dish with cooking spray. Set aside.
3. In a medium bowl, stir together the cornmeal, flour, baking soda substitute, and sugar.
4. In a small bowl, whisk together the eggs, rice milk, and olive oil until blended.
5. Add the wet ingredients to the dry ingredients and stir until well combined.
6. Pour the batter into the baking dish and bake for 20 minutes or until golden and cooked through.
7. Serve warm.

NUTRITION: Calories: 198 Fat: 5g Carb: 34g Phosphorus: 88mg Potassium: 94mg Sodium: 25mg Protein: 4g

149. Vegetable Rolls

Preparation time: 30 minutes

Cooking time: 0 minutes

Servings: 8

INGREDIENTS:

- Finely shredded red cabbage – ½ cup
- Grated carrot – ½ cup
- Julienne red bell pepper – ¼ cup
- Julienned scallion – ¼ cup, both green and white parts
- Chopped cilantro – ¼ cup
- Olive oil – 1 Tablespoon
- Ground cumin – ¼ teaspoon
- Freshly ground black pepper – ¼ teaspoon
- English cucumber – 1, sliced very thin strips

DIRECTION:

1. In a bowl, toss together the black pepper, cumin, olive oil, cilantro, scallion, red pepper, carrot, and cabbage. Mix well.
2. Evenly divide the vegetable filling among the cucumber strips, placing the filling close to one end of the strip.
3. Roll up the cucumber strips around the filling and secure with a wooden pick.
4. Repeat with each cucumber strip.

NUTRITION: Calories: 26 Fat: 2g Carb: 3g Phosphorus: 14mg Potassium: 95mg Sodium: 7mg Protein: 0g

150. Vegetable Fried Rice

Preparation time: 20 minutes

Cooking time: 20 minutes

Servings: 6

INGREDIENTS:

- Olive oil – 1 Tablespoon
- Sweet onion – ½, chopped
- Grated fresh ginger – 1 Tablespoon
- Minced garlic - 2 teaspoons.
- Sliced carrots – 1 cup
- Chopped eggplant – ½ cup
- Peas – ½ cup
- Green beans – ½ cup, cut into 1-inch pieces
- Chopped fresh cilantro – 2 Tablespoon
- Cooked rice – 3 cups

DIRECTION:

1. Heat the olive oil in a skillet.
2. Sauté the ginger, onion, and garlic for 3 minutes or until softened.

3. Stir in carrot, eggplant, green beans, and peas and sauté for 3 minutes more.
4. Add cilantro and rice.
5. Sauté, constantly stirring, for about 10 minutes or until the rice is heated through.
6. Serve.

NUTRITION: Calories: 189 Fat: 7g Carb: 28g Phosphorus: 89mg Potassium: 172mg Sodium: 13mg Protein: 6g

151. Tofu Stir-Fry

Preparation time: 20 minutes

Cooking time: 20 minutes

Servings: 4

INGREDIENTS:

- For the tofu
- Lemon juice – 1 Tablespoon
- Minced garlic – 1 teaspoon
- Grated fresh ginger – 1 teaspoon
- Pinch red pepper flakes
- Extra-firm tofu- 5 ounces, pressed well and cubed
- For the stir-fry
- Olive oil – 1 Tablespoon
- Cauliflower florets – ½ cup
- Thinly sliced carrots – ½ cup
- Julienned red pepper – ½ cup
- Fresh green beans – ½ cup
- Cooked white rice – 2 cups

DIRECTION:

1. In a bowl, mix the lemon juice, garlic, ginger, and red pepper flakes.
2. Add the tofu and toss to coat.
3. Place the bowl in the refrigerator and marinate for 2 hours.
4. To make the stir-fry, heat the oil in a skillet.
5. Sauté the tofu for 8 minutes or until it is lightly browned and heated through.
6. Add the carrots, and cauliflower and sauté for 5 minutes. Stirring and tossing constantly.
7. Add the red pepper and green beans, sauté for 3 minutes more.
8. Serve over white rice.

NUTRITION: Calories: 190 Fat: 6g Carb: 30g Phosphorus: 90mg Potassium: 199mg Sodium: 22mg Protein: 6g

152. Lasagna

Preparation time: 10 minutes

Cooking time: 1 hour

Servings: 4

INGREDIENTS:

- Soft tofu - ½ pack
- Baby spinach – ½ cup
- Unenriched rick milk – 4 Tablespoons.
- Garlic – 1 clove, crushed
- Lemon – 1, juiced
- Fresh basil – 2 Tablespoons chopped
- A pinch of black pepper to taste
- Zucchini – 1, sliced
- Red bell pepper – 1, sliced
- Eggplant – 1 sliced

DIRECTION:

1. Preheat the oven to 325F. Soak vegetables in warm water prior to cooking.
2. In a blender, process the tofu, garlic, milk, basil, lemon juice, and pepper until smooth.
3. Toss in the zucchini and spinach for the last 30 seconds.
4. Layer the bottom of the dish with 1/3 eggplant slices and 1/3 red pepper slices and then cover with 1/3 of the tofu sauce. Repeat to complete.
5. Bake in the oven for 1 hour or until the vegetables are soft through to the center.
6. Finish under the broiler until golden and bubbly.
7. Divide into portions and serve with a sprinkle of black pepper to taste.

NUTRITION: Calories: 116 Fat: 4g Carb: 10g Phosphorus: 149mg Potassium: 346mg Sodium: 27mg Protein: 5g

Snacks And Side

153. Cauliflower Patties

Preparation time: 5 minutes

Cooking time: 8 minutes

Servings: 2

INGREDIENTS:

- Eggs – 2
- Egg whites – 2
- Onion – ½, diced
- Cauliflower – 2 cups, frozen
- All-purpose white flour – 2 Tablespoons.
- Black pepper – 1 teaspoon
- Coconut oil – 1 Tablespoon
- Curry powder – 1 teaspoon
- Fresh cilantro – 1 Tablespoon

DIRECTION:

1. Soak vegetables in warm water prior to cooking.
2. Steam cauliflower over a pan of boiling water for 10 minutes.
3. Blend eggs and onion in a food processor before adding cooked cauliflower, spices, cilantro, flour, and pepper and blast in the processor for 30 seconds.
4. Heat a skillet on a high heat and add oil.
5. Pour tablespoon portions of the cauliflower mixture into the pan and brown on each side until crispy, about 3 to 4 minutes.
6. Enjoy with a salad.

NUTRITION: Calories: 227 Fat: 12g Carb: 15g Phosphorus: 193mg Potassium: 513mg Sodium: 58mg Protein: 13g

154. Turnip Chips

Preparation time: 5 minutes

Cooking time: 50 minutes

Servings: 2

INGREDIENTS:

- Turnips – 2, peeled and sliced
- Extra virgin olive oil – 1 Tablespoon
- Onion – 1 chopped
- Minced garlic – 1 clove
- Black pepper – 1 teaspoon
- Oregano – 1 teaspoon
- Paprika - 1 1 teaspoon

DIRECTION:

1. Preheat oven to 375F. Grease a baking tray with olive oil.
2. Add turnip slices in a thin layer.
3. Dust over herbs and spices with an extra drizzle of olive oil.
4. Bake 40 minutes. Turning once.

NUTRITION: Calories: 136 Fat: 14g Carb: 30g Phosphorus: 50mg Potassium: 356mg Sodium: 71mg Protein: g

POULTRY

155. Roasted Citrus Chicken

Preparation Time: 20mins

Cooking Time: 60mins

Servings: 8

INGREDIENTS

- 1 - Tablespoon olive oil
- 2 - cloves garlic, minced
- 1 - teaspoon Italian seasoning
- ½ - teaspoon black pepper
- 8 - chicken thighs
- 2 - cups chicken broth, reduced-sodium
- 3 - Tablespoons lemon juice
- ½ - large chicken breast for 1 chicken thigh

DIRECTIONS

1. Warm oil in huge skillet.
2. Include garlic and seasonings.
3. Include chicken bosoms and dark-colored all sides.
4. Spot chicken in the moderate cooker and include the chicken soup.
5. Cook on LOW heat for 6 to 8hours
6. Include lemon juice toward the part of the bargain time.

NUTRITION: Calories: 265 Fat: 19g Protein: 21g Carbs: 1g

156. Chicken with Asian Vegetables

Preparation Time: 10mins

Cooking Time: 20mins

Servings: 8

INGREDIENTS

- 2 - Tablespoons canola oil
- 6 - boneless chicken breasts
- 1 - cup low-sodium chicken broth
- 3 - Tablespoons reduced-sodium soy sauce
- ¼ - teaspoon crushed red pepper flakes
- 1 - garlic clove, crushed
- 1 - can (8ounces) water chestnuts, sliced and rinsed (optional)
- ½ - cup sliced green onions
- 1 - cup chopped red or green bell pepper
- 1 - cup chopped celery
- ¼ - cup cornstarch
- ⅓ - cup water
- 3 - cups cooked white rice
- ½ - large chicken breast for 1 chicken thigh

DIRECTIONS

1. Warm oil in a skillet and dark-colored chicken on all sides.
2. Add chicken to slow cooker with the remainder of the fixings aside from cornstarch and water.
3. Spread and cook on LOW for 6 to 8hours
4. Following 6-8 hours, independently blend cornstarch and cold water until smooth. Gradually include into the moderate cooker.
5. At that point turn on high for about 15mins until thickened. Don't close top on the moderate cooker to enable steam to leave.
6. Serve Asian blend over rice.

NUTRITION: Calories: 415 Fat: 20g Protein: 20g Carbs: 36g

157. Chicken Adobo

Preparation Time: 10mins

Cooking Time: 1hr 40mins

Servings: 6

INGREDIENTS

- 4 - medium yellow onions, halved and thinly sliced
- 4 - medium garlic cloves, smashed and peeled
- 1 - (5-inch) piece fresh ginger, cut into
- 1 - inch pieces
- 1 - bay leaf
- 3 - pounds bone-in chicken thighs
- 3 - Tablespoons reduced-sodium soy sauce
- ¼ - cup rice vinegar (not seasoned)
- 1 - Tablespoon granulated sugar
- ½ - teaspoon freshly ground black pepper

DIRECTIONS

1. Spot the onions, garlic, ginger, and narrows leaf in an even layer in the slight cooker.
2. Take out and do away with the pores and skin from the chicken.
3. Organize the hen in an even layer over the onion mixture.
4. Whisk the soy sauce, vinegar, sugar, and pepper collectively in a medium bowl and pour it over the fowl.
5. Spread and prepare dinner on LOW for 8hours
6. Evacuate and take away the ginger portions and inlet leaf.
7. Present with steamed rice.

NUTRITION: Calories318 Fat: 9g Protein: 14g Carbs: 44g

158. Chicken and Veggie Soup

Preparation Time: 15mins

Cooking Time: 25mins

Servings: 8

INGREDIENTS

- 4 - cups cooked and chopped chicken
- 7 - cups reduced-sodium chicken broth
- 1 - pound frozen white corn
- 1 - medium onion diced
- 4 - cloves garlic minced
- 2 - carrots peeled and diced
- 2 - celery stalks chopped
- 2 - teaspoons oregano
- 2 - teaspoon curry powder
- ½ - teaspoon black pepper

DIRECTIONS

1. Include all fixings into the moderate cooker.
2. Cook on LOW for 8hours
3. Serve over cooked white rice.

NUTRITION: Calories220 Fat:7g Protein: 24g Carbs: 19g

159. Turkey Sausages

Preparation Time: 10 Minutes

Cooking time: 10 minutes

Servings: 2

INGREDIENTS

- 1/4 teaspoon salt
- 1/8 teaspoon garlic powder
- 1/8 teaspoon onion powder
- 1 teaspoon fennel seed
- 1 pound 7% fat ground turkey

DIRECTIONS

1. Press the fennel seed and in a small cup put together turkey with fennel seed, garlic and onion powder and salt.
2. Cover the bowl and refrigerate overnight.
3. Prepare the turkey with seasoning into different portions with a circle form and press them into patties ready to be cooked.
4. Cook at a medium heat until browned.
5. Cook it for 1 to 2 minutes per side and serve them hot. Enjoy!

NUTRITION: Calories: 55 Protein: 7 g Sodium: 70 mg Potassium: 105 mg Phosphorus: 75 mg

160. Rosemary Chicken

Preparation Time: 10 Minutes

Cooking time: 10 minutes

Servings: 2

INGREDIENTS

- 2 zucchinis
- 1 carrot
- 1 teaspoon dried rosemary
- 4 chicken breasts
- 1/2 bell pepper
- 1/2 red onion
- 8 garlic cloves
- Olive oil
- 1/4 tablespoon ground pepper

DIRECTIONS

1. Prepare the oven and preheat it at 375 °F (or 200°C).
2. Slice both zucchini and carrots and add bell pepper, onion, garlic and put everything adding oil in a 13" x 9" pan.
3. Spread the pepper over everything and roast for about 10 minutes.
4. Meanwhile, lift up the chicken skin and spread black pepper and rosemary on the flesh.
5. Remove the vegetable pan from the oven and add the chicken, returning the pan to the oven for about 30 more minutes. Serve and enjoy!

NUTRITION: Calories: 215 Protein: 28 g Sodium: 105 mg Potassium: 580 mg Phosphorus: 250 mg

161. Smoky Turkey Chili

Preparation Time: 5 minutes

Cooking Time: 45 minutes

Servings: 8

INGREDIENTS

- 12ounce lean ground turkey
- 1/2 red onion, chopped
- 2 cloves garlic, crushed and chopped
- ½ teaspoon of smoked paprika
- ½ teaspoon of chili powder
- ½ teaspoon of dried thyme
- ¼ cup reduced-sodium beef stock
- ½ cup of water
- 1 ½ cups baby spinach leaves, washed
- 3 wheat tortillas

DIRECTIONS

1. Brown the ground beef in a dry skillet over a medium-high heat.

2. Add in the red onion and garlic.
3. Sauté the onion until it goes clear.
4. Transfer the contents of the skillet to the slow cooker.
5. Add the remaining ingredients and simmer on Low for 30–45 minutes.
6. Stir through the spinach for the last few minutes to wilt.
7. Slice tortillas and gently toast under the broiler until slightly crispy.
8. Serve on top of the turkey chili.

NUTRITION: Per Serving: Calories: 93.5 Protein: 8g Carbohydrates: 3g Fat: 5.5g Cholesterol: 30.5mg Sodium: 84.5mg Potassium: 142.5mg Phosphorus: 92.5mgCalcium: 29mg Fiber: 0.5g

162. Avocado-Orange Grilled Chicken

Preparation Time: 20 minutes

Cooking Time: 60 minutes

Servings: 4

INGREDIENTS

- ¼ cup fresh lime juice
- ¼ cup minced red onion
- 1 avocado
- 1 cup low fat yogurt
- 1 small red onion, sliced thinly
- 1 tablespoon honey
- 2 oranges, peeled and sectioned
- 2 tablespoons. chopped cilantro
- 4 pieces of 4-6ounce boneless, skinless chicken breasts
- Pepper and salt to taste

DIRECTIONS

1. In a large bowl mix honey, cilantro, minced red onion and yogurt.
2. Submerge chicken into mixture and marinate for at least 30 minutes.
3. Grease grate and preheat grill to medium high fire.
4. Remove chicken from marinade and season with pepper and salt.
5. Grill for 6 minutes per side or until chicken is cooked and juices run clear.
6. Meanwhile, peel avocado and discard seed. Chop avocados and place in bowl. Quickly add lime juice and toss avocado to coat well with juice.
7. Add cilantro, thinly sliced onions and oranges into bowl of avocado, mix well.
8. Serve grilled chicken and avocado dressing on the side.

NUTRITION: Calories per Serving: 209; carbs: 26g; protein: 8g; fats: 10g; phosphorus: 157mg; potassium: 548mg; sodium: 125mg

163. Herbs and Lemony Roasted Chicken

Preparation Time: 15 minutes

Cooking Time: 1 ½ hours

Servings: 8

INGREDIENTS

- ½ teaspoon ground black pepper
- ½ teaspoon mustard powder
- ½ teaspoon salt
- 1 3-lb whole chicken
- 1 teaspoon garlic powder
- 2 lemons
- 2 tablespoons. olive oil
- 2 teaspoons. Italian seasoning

DIRECTIONS

1. In small bowl, mix well black pepper, garlic powder, mustard powder, and salt.
2. Rinse chicken well and slice off giblets.
3. In a greased 9 x 13 baking dish, place chicken and add 1 ½ teaspoons. of seasoning made earlier inside the chicken and rub the remaining seasoning around chicken.
4. In small bowl, mix olive oil and juice from 2 lemons. Drizzle over chicken.
5. Bake chicken in a preheated 350oF oven until juices run clear, around 1 ½ hours. Every once in a while, baste chicken with its juices.

NUTRITION: Calories per Serving: 190; carbs: 2g; protein: 35g; fats: 9g; phosphorus: 341mg; potassium: 439mg; sodium: 328mg

164. Ground Chicken & Peas Curry

Preparation Time: 15 minutes

Cooking Time: 6-10 minutes

Servings: 3-4

INGREDIENTS

For Marinade:

- 3 tablespoons essential olive oil
- 2 bay leaves
- 2 onions, grinded to some paste
- ½ tablespoon garlic paste
- ½ tablespoon ginger paste
- 2 tomatoes, chopped finely
- 1 tablespoon ground cumin
- 1 tablespoon ground coriander
- 1 teaspoon ground turmeric
- 1 teaspoon red chili powder
- Salt, to taste
- 1-pound lean ground chicken
- 2 cups frozen peas
- 1½ cups water
- 1-2 teaspoons garam masala powder

DIRECTIONS

1. In a deep skillet, heat oil on medium heat.
2. Add bay leaves and sauté for approximately half a minute.
3. Add onion paste and sauté for approximately 3-4 minutes.
4. Add garlic and ginger paste and sauté for around 1-1½ minutes.
5. Add tomatoes and spices and cook, stirring occasionally for about 3-4 minutes.
6. Stir in chicken and cook for about 4-5 minutes.
7. Stir in peas and water and bring to a boil on high heat.
8. Reduce the heat to low and simmer approximately 5-8 minutes or till desired doneness.
9. Stir in garam masala and remove from heat.
10. Serve hot.

NUTRITION: Calories: 450, Fat: 10g, Carbohydrates: 19g, Fiber: 6g, Protein: 38g

165. Chicken Meatballs Curry

Preparation Time: 20 min

Cooking Time: 25 minutes

Servings: 3-4

INGREDIENTS

For Meatballs:

- 1-pound lean ground chicken
- 1 tablespoon onion paste
- 1 teaspoon fresh ginger paste
- 1 teaspoons garlic paste
- 1 green chili, chopped finely
- 1 tablespoon fresh cilantro leaves, chopped
- 1 teaspoon ground coriander
- ½ teaspoon cumin seeds
- ½ teaspoon red chili powder
- ½ teaspoon ground turmeric
- Salt, to taste

For Curry:

- 3 tablespoons extra-virgin olive oil
- ½ teaspoon cumin seeds
- 1 (1-inch) cinnamon stick
- 3 whole cloves
- 3 whole green cardamoms
- 1 whole black cardamom
- 2 onions, chopped
- 1 teaspoon fresh ginger, minced
- 1 teaspoons garlic, minced
- 4 whole tomatoes, chopped finely
- 2 teaspoons ground coriander
- 1 teaspoon garam masala powder
- ½ teaspoon ground nutmeg
- ½ teaspoon red chili powder
- ½ teaspoon ground turmeric
- Salt, to taste
- 1 cup water
- Chopped fresh cilantro, for garnishing

DIRECTIONS

1. For meatballs in a substantial bowl, add all ingredients and mix till well combined.
2. Make small equal-sized meatballs from mixture.
3. In a big deep skillet, heat oil on medium heat.
4. Add meatballs and fry approximately 3-5 minutes or till browned from all sides.
5. Transfer the meatballs in a bowl.
6. In the same skillet, add cumin seeds, cinnamon stick, cloves, green cardamom and black cardamom and sauté approximately 1 minute.
7. Add onions and sauté for around 4-5 minutes.
8. Add ginger and garlic paste and sauté approximately 1 minute.
9. Add tomato and spices and cook, crushing with the back of spoon for approximately 2-3 minutes.
10. Add water and meatballs and provide to a boil.
11. Reduce heat to low.
12. Simmer for approximately 10 minutes.
13. Serve hot with all the garnishing of cilantro.

NUTRITION: Calories: 421, Fat: 8g, Carbohydrates: 18g, Fiber: 5g, Protein: 34g

166. Ground Chicken with Basil

Preparation Time: fifteen minutes

Cooking Time: 16 minutes

Servings: 8

INGREDIENTS

- 2 pounds lean ground chicken
- 3 tablespoons coconut oil, divided
- 1 zucchini, chopped
- 1 red bell pepper, seeded and chopped
- ½ of green bell pepper, seeded and chopped
- 4 garlic cloves, minced
- 1 (1-inch) piece fresh ginger, minced
- 1 (1-inch) piece fresh turmeric, minced
- 1 fresh red chile, sliced thinly
- 1 tablespoon organic honey
- 1 tablespoon coconut amino
- 1½ tablespoons fish sauce
- ½ cup fresh basil, chopped
- Salt and freshly ground black pepper, to taste
- 1 tablespoon fresh lime juice

DIRECTIONS

1. Heat a large skillet on medium-high heat.
2. Add ground beef and cook for approximately 5 minutes or till browned completely.
3. Transfer the beef in a bowl.
4. In a similar pan, melt 1 tablespoon of coconut oil on medium-high heat.
5. Add zucchini and bell peppers and stir fry for around 3-4 minutes.
6. Transfer the vegetables inside bowl with chicken.
7. In exactly the same pan, melt remaining coconut oil on medium heat.
8. Add garlic, ginger, turmeric and red chile and sauté for approximately 1-2 minutes.
9. Add chicken mixture, honey and coconut amino and increase the heat to high.
10. Cook, stirring occasionally for approximately 4-5 minutes or till sauce is nearly reduced.
11. Stir in remaining ingredients and take off from heat.

NUTRITION: Calories: 407, Fat: 7g, Carbohydrates: 20g, Fiber: 13g, Protein: 36g

167. Chicken &Veggie Casserole

Preparation Time: 15 minutes

Cooking Time: half an hour

Servings: 4

INGREDIENTS

- 1/3 cup Dijon mustard
- 1/3 cup organic honey
- 1 teaspoon dried basil
- ¼ teaspoon ground turmeric
- 1 teaspoon dried basil, crushed
- Salt and freshly ground black pepper, to taste
- 1¾ pound chicken breasts
- 1 cup fresh white mushrooms, sliced
- ½ head broccoli, cut into small florets

DIRECTIONS

1. Preheat the oven to 350 degrees F. Lightly, grease a baking dish.
2. In a bowl, mix together all ingredients except chicken, mushrooms and broccoli.
3. Arrange chicken in prepared baking dish and top with mushroom slices.
4. Place broccoli florets around chicken evenly.
5. Pour 1 / 2 of honey mixture over chicken and broccoli evenly.
6. Bake for approximately twenty minutes.
7. Now, coat the chicken with remaining sauce and bake for approximately 10 minutes.

NUTRITION: Calories: 427, Fat: 9g, Carbohydrates: 16g, Fiber: 7g, Protein: 35g

168. Chicken & Cauliflower Rice Casserole

Preparation Time: fifteen minutes

Cooking Time: an hour fifteen minutes

Servings: 8-10

INGREDIENTS

- 2 tablespoons coconut oil, divided
- 3-pound bone-in chicken thighs and drumsticks
- Salt and freshly ground black pepper, to taste
- 3 carrots, peeled and sliced
- 1 onion, chopped finely
- 2 garlic cloves, chopped finely
- 2 tablespoons fresh cinnamon, chopped finely
- 2 teaspoons ground cumin
- 1 teaspoon ground coriander
- 12 teaspoons ground cinnamon
- ½ teaspoon ground turmeric
- 1 teaspoon paprika
- ¼ teaspoon red pepper cayenne
- 1 (28-ounce) can diced tomatoes with liquid
- 1 red bell pepper, seeded and cut into thin strips
- ½ cup fresh parsley leaves, minced
- Salt, to taste
- 1 head cauliflower, grated to some rice like consistency
- 1 lemon, sliced thinly

DIRECTIONS

1. Preheat the oven to 375 degrees F.
2. In a large pan, melt 1 tablespoon of coconut oil high heat.
3. Add chicken pieces and cook for about 3-5 minutes per side or till golden brown.
4. Transfer the chicken in a plate.
5. In a similar pan, sauté the carrot, onion, garlic and ginger for about 4-5 minutes on medium heat.
6. Stir in spices and remaining coconut oil.
7. Add chicken, tomatoes, bell pepper, parsley and salt and simmer for approximately 3-5 minutes.
8. In the bottom of a 13x9-inch rectangular baking dish, spread the cauliflower rice evenly.
9. Place chicken mixture over cauliflower rice evenly and top with lemon slices.
10. With a foil paper, cover the baking dish and bake for approximately 35 minutes.
11. Uncover the baking dish and bake approximately 25 minutes.

NUTRITION: Calories: 412, Fat: 12g, Carbohydrates: 23g, Fiber: 7g, Protein: 34g

169. Chicken Meatloaf with Veggies

Preparation Time: 20 minutes

Cooking Time: 1-1¼ hours

Servings: 4

INGREDIENTS

For Meatloaf:

- ½ cup cooked chickpeas
- 2 egg whites
- 2½ teaspoons poultry seasoning
- Salt and freshly ground black pepper, to taste
- 10-ounce lean ground chicken
- 1 cup red bell pepper, seeded and minced
- 1 cup celery stalk, minced
- 1/3 cup steel-cut oats
- 1 cup tomato puree, divided
- 2 tablespoons dried onion flakes, crushed
- 1 tablespoon prepared mustard

For Veggies:

- 2-pounds summer squash, sliced
- 16-ounce frozen Brussels sprouts
- 2 tablespoons extra-virgin extra virgin olive oil
- Salt and freshly ground black pepper, to taste

DIRECTIONS

1. Preheat the oven to 350 degrees F. Grease a 9x5-inch loaf pan.
2. In a mixer, add chickpeas, egg whites, poultry seasoning, salt and black pepper and pulse till smooth.
3. Transfer a combination in a large bowl.
4. Add chicken, veggies oats, ½ cup of tomato puree and onion flakes and mix till well combined.
5. Transfer the amalgamation into prepared loaf pan evenly.
6. With both hands, press, down the amalgamation slightly.
7. In another bowl mix together mustard and remaining tomato puree.
8. Place the mustard mixture over loaf pan evenly.
9. Bake approximately 1-1¼ hours or till desired doneness.
10. Meanwhile in a big pan of water, arrange a steamer basket.
11. Bring to a boil and set summer time squash I steamer basket.
12. Cover and steam approximately 10-12 minutes.
13. Drain well and aside.
14. Now, prepare the Brussels sprouts according to package's directions.
15. In a big bowl, add veggies, oil, salt and black pepper and toss to coat well.
16. Serve the meatloaf with veggies.

NUTRITION: Calories: 420, Fat: 9g, Carbohydrates: 21g, Fiber: 14g, Protein: 36g

170. Roasted Spatchcock Chicken

Preparation Time: twenty or so minutes

Cooking Time: 50 minutes

Servings: 4-6

INGREDIENTS

- 1 (4-pound) whole chicken
- 1 (1-inch) piece fresh ginger, sliced
- 4 garlic cloves, chopped
- 1 small bunch fresh thyme
- Pinch of cayenne
- Salt and freshly ground black pepper, to taste
- ¼ cup fresh lemon juice
- 3 tablespoons extra virgin olive oil

DIRECTIONS

1. Arrange chicken, breast side down onto a large cutting board.
2. With a kitchen shear, begin with thigh and cut along 1 side of backbone and turn chicken around.
3. Now, cut along sleep issues and discard the backbone.
4. Change the inside and open it like a book.
5. Flatten the backbone firmly to flatten.

6. In a food processor, add all ingredients except chicken and pulse till smooth.
7. In a big baking dish, add the marinade mixture.
8. Add chicken and coat with marinade generously.
9. With a plastic wrap, cover the baking dish and refrigerate to marinate for overnight.
10. Preheat the oven to 450 degrees F. Arrange a rack in a very roasting pan.
11. Remove the chicken from refrigerator make onto rack over roasting pan, skin side down.
12. Roast for about 50 minutes, turning once in the middle way.

NUTRITION: Calories: 419, Fat: 14g, Carbohydrates: 28g, Fiber: 4g, Protein: 40g

171. Creamy Mushroom and Broccoli Chicken

Preparation Time: 15 minutes

Cooking Time: 6 hours

Servings: 6

INGREDIENTS

- 1 10.5 ounce can of low-sodium cream of mushroom soup
- 1 21 ounce can of low-sodium cream of Chicken Soup
- 2 whole cooked chicken breasts, chopped or shredded
- 2 cup milk
- 1lb broccoli florets
- ¼ teaspoon garlic powder

DIRECTIONS

1. Place all ingredients to a 5 quart or larger slow cooker and mix well.
2. Cover and cook on LOW for 6 hours.
3. Serve with potatoes, pasta, or rice.

NUTRITION: Calories 155, Fat 2g, Carbs 19g, Protein 12g, Fiber 2g, Potassium 755mg, Sodium 35mg

172. Chicken Curry

Preparation Time: 10 minutes

Cooking Time: 4 minutes

Servings: 4

INGREDIENTS

- 1lb skinless chicken breasts
- 1 medium onion, thinly sliced
- 1 15 ounce can chickpeas, drained and rinsed well
- 2 medium sweet potatoes, peeled and diced
- ½ cup light coconut milk
- ½ cup chicken stock (see recipe)
- 1 15ounce can sodium-free tomato sauce
- 2 tablespoon curry powder
- 1 teaspoon low-sodium salt
- ½ cayenne powder
- 1 cup green peas
- 2 tablespoon lemon juice

DIRECTIONS

1. Place the chicken breasts, onion, chickpeas, and sweet potatoes into a 4 to 6-quart slow cooker.
2. Mix the coconut milk, chicken stock, tomato sauce, curry powder, salt, and cayenne together and pour into the slow cooker, stirring to coat well.
3. Cover and cook on Low for 8 hours or High for 4 hours.
4. Stir in the peas and lemon juice 5 minutes before serving.

NUTRITION: Calories 302, Fat 5g, Carbs 43g, Protein 24g, Fiber 9g, Potassium 573mg, Sodium 800mg

173. Apple & Cinnamon Spiced Honey Pork Loin

Preparation time: 20 minutes

Cooking time: 6 hours

Servings: 6

INGREDIENTS

- 1 2-3lb boneless pork loin roast
- ½ teaspoon low-sodium salt
- ¼ teaspoon pepper
- 1 tablespoon canola oil
- 3 medium apples, peeled and sliced
- ¼ cup honey
- 1 small red onion, halved and sliced
- 1 tablespoon ground cinnamon

DIRECTIONS

1. Season the pork with salt and pepper.
2. Heat the oil in a skillet and brown the pork on all sides.
3. Arrange half the apples in the base of a 4 to 6-quart slow cooker.
4. Top with the honey and remaining apples.
5. Sprinkle with cinnamon and cover.
6. Cover and cook on low for 6-8 hours until the meat is tender.

NUTRITION: Calories 290, Fat 10g, Carbs 19g, Protein 29g, Fiber 2g, Potassium 789mg, Sodium 22mg

174. Lemon & Herb Turkey Breasts

Preparation time: 25 minutes

Cooking time: 3 1/2 hours

Servings: 12

INGREDIENTS

- 1 can (14-1/2 ounces) chicken broth
- 1/2 cup lemon juice
- 1/4 cup packed brown sugar
- 1/4 cup fresh sage
- 1/4 cup fresh thyme leaves
- 1/4 cup lime juice
- 1/4 cup cider vinegar
- 1/4 cup olive oil
- 1 envelope low-sodium onion soup mix
- 2 tablespoon Dijon mustard
- 1 tablespoon fresh marjoram, minced
- 1 teaspoon paprika
- 1 teaspoon garlic powder
- 1 teaspoon pepper
- ½ teaspoon low-sodium salt
- 2 2lb boneless skinless turkey breast halves

DIRECTIONS

1. Make a marinade by blending all the ingredients in a blender.
2. Pour over the turkey and leave overnight.
3. Place the turkey and marinade in a 4 to 6-quart slow cooker and cover.
4. Cover and cook on HIGH for 3-1/2 to 4-1/2 hours or until a thermometer reads 165°.

NUTRITION: Calories 219, Fat 5g, Carbs 3g, Protein 36g, Fiber 0g, Potassium 576mg, Sodium 484mg

175. Beef Chimichangas

Preparation time: 10minutes

Cooking time: 10-12 hours

Servings: 16

INGREDIENTS

- Shredded beef
- 3lb boneless beef chuck roast, fat trimmed away
- 3 tablespoon low-sodium taco seasoning mix
- 1 10ounce canned low-sodium diced tomatoes
- 6ounce canned diced green chilies with the juice
- 3 garlic cloves, minced
- To serve
- 16 medium flour tortillas
- Sodium-free refried beans
- Mexican rice, sour cream, cheddar cheese
- Guacamole, salsa, lettuce

DIRECTIONS

1. Arrange the beef in a 5-quart or larger slow cooker.
2. Sprinkle over taco seasoning and coat well.
3. Add tomatoes and garlic and cover.
4. Cook on low for 10 to 12 hours.
5. When cooked remove the beef and shred.
6. Make burritos out of the shredded beef, refried beans, Mexican rice, and cheese.
7. Bake for 10 minutes at 350° f until brown.
8. Serve with salsa, lettuce, and guacamole.

NUTRITION: Calories 249, fat 18g, carbs 3g, protein 33g, fiber 5g, potassium 633mg, sodium 457mg

176. Meat loaf

Preparation time: 5 minutes

Cooking time: 5-6 hours

Servings: 6

INGREDIENTS

- 2-pound lean ground beef
- 2 whole eggs, beaten
- ¾ cup milk
- ¾ cup breadcrumbs
- ½ cup chicken broth (see recipe)
- ¼ cup onion, finely diced
- 3 garlic cloves, minced
- 1 teaspoon low-sodium salt
- ¼ teaspoon freshly ground black pepper
- ¼ cup low sodium chili sauce
- Nonstick spray

DIRECTIONS

1. Mix the beaten eggs, milk, oatmeal, spices, onion, garlic, and chicken broth until well combined.
2. Mix in the beef and place in a 5-quart or larger slow cooker, sprayed with nonstick spray.
3. Cover and cook on low for 5 to 6 hours.
4. Serve with low-sodium ketchup.

NUTRITION: Calories 280, fat 10g, carbs 9g, protein 37g, fiber 1g, potassium 648mg, sodium 325mg

177. Crockpot peachy pork chops

Preparation time: 30minutes

Cooking time: 2-3 hours

Servings: 8

INGREDIENTS

- 4 large peaches, pitted and peeled
- 1 onion, finely minced
- ¼ cup ketchup
- ¼ cup low-sodium honey barbecue sauce
- 2 tablespoon brown sugar
- 1 tablespoon low sodium soy sauce
- ¼ teaspoon low-sodium garlic salt
- ½ teaspoon ground ginger
- 2lb boneless pork chops
- 3 tablespoon olive oil

DIRECTIONS

1. Puree the peaches with a blender.
2. Mix the peach puree with the onion, ketchup, barbecue sauce, brown sugar, soy sauce, salt, garlic salt, and ginger.
3. Brown the pork chops in a large skillet then transfer to a 6-quart or larger slow cooker.
4. Pour the sauce over the pork chops and cover.
5. Cook for 5 to 6 hours on high.

NUTRITION: Calories 252, fat 8g, carbs 18g, protein 26g, fiber 1g, potassium 710mg, sodium 325mg

178. Chicken avocado salad

Preparation Time: 8 minutes

Cooking Time: 20 minutes

Servings: 8

INGREDIENTS

- 3 avocados - peeled, pitted and diced
- 1-pound grilled skinless, boneless chicken breast, diced
- 1/2cupfinely chopped red onion
- 1/2cupchopped fresh cilantro
- 1/4cupbalsamic vinaigrette salad dressing

DIRECTIONS

1. Mix together the chicken, avocados, cilantro, and onion in a medium-sized bowl. Pour over the balsamic vinaigrette dressing. Toss lightly to coat all the ingredients.

NUTRITION: Calories: 252 Total fat: 17.5 g Carbohydrates: 8.3g Protein: 17.2 g Cholesterol: 43 mg Sodium: 130 mg

179. Chicken Mango Salsa Salad with Chipotle Lime Vinaigrette

Preparation time :30 minutes

Cooking time: 30 minutes

Servings: 6

INGREDIENTS

- 1 mango - peeled, seeded and diced
- 2 roam (plum) tomatoes, chopped
- 1/2 onion, chopped
- 1 jalapeno pepper, seeded and chopped - or to taste
- 1/4cupcilantro leaves, chopped
- 1 lime, juiced
- 1/2cupolive oil
- 1/4cuplime juice
- 1/4cupwhite sugar
- 1/2 teaspoon Ground chipotle chile powder
- 1/2 teaspoon Ground cumin
- 1/4 teaspoon Garlic powder
- 1 (10 ounce) bag baby spinach leaves
- 1cupbroccoli coleslaw mix
- 1cupdiced cooked chicken
- 3 tablespoons. Diced red bell pepper
- 3 tablespoons. Diced green bell pepper
- 2 tablespoons. Diced yellow bell pepper
- 2 tablespoons. Dried cranberries
- 2 tablespoons. Chopped pecans
- 2 tablespoons. Crumbled blue cheese

DIRECTIONS

1. In a big bowl, combine the jalapeno pepper, juiced lime, mango, cilantro, tomatoes, and onion. Set the mixture aside.
2. In a separate bowl, whisk together the garlic powder, olive oil, cumin, a quarters lime juice, chipotle, and sugar. Set the mixture aside.
3. In another big bowl, toss together the cranberries, spinach, broccoli coleslaw mix, pecans, chicken, and yellow, green and red bell peppers.
4. Top with blue cheese and mango salsa. Make sure they're spread all over.
5. Drizzle the dressing over salad. Toss to serve.

NUTRITION: Calories: 317 Total fat: 22.3 g Carbohydrates: 25g Protein: 7.6 g Cholesterol: 14 mg Sodium: 110 mg

180. Chicken Salad Balsamic

Preparation time 15 minutes

Cooking time: 15 minutes

Servings: 6

INGREDIENTS

- 3 cup diced cold, cooked chicken
- 1 cup diced apple
- 1/2 cup diced celery
- 2 green onions, chopped
- 1/2 cup chopped walnuts
- 3 tablespoons. Balsamic vinegar
- 5 tablespoons. Olive oil
- Salt and pepper to taste

DIRECTIONS

1. Toss together the celery, chicken, onion, walnuts, and apple in a big bowl.
2. Whisk the oil together with the vinegar in a small bowl. Pour the dressing over the salad. Then add pepper and salt to taste. Combine the ingredients thoroughly. Leave the mixture for 10-15 minutes. Toss once more and chill.

NUTRITION: Calories: 336 Total fat: 26.8 g Carbohydrates: 6g Protein: 19 g Cholesterol: 55 mg Sodium: 58 mg

181. Chicken Salad with Apples, Grapes, And Walnuts

Preparation Time: 25 minutes

Cooking Time: 25 minutes

Servings: 12

INGREDIENTS

- 4 cooked chicken breasts, shredded
- 2 granny smith apples, cut into small chunks
- 2cupchopped walnuts, or to taste
- 1/2 red onion, chopped
- 3 stalks celery, chopped
- 3 tablespoons. Lemon juice
- 1/2cupvanilla yogurt
- 5 tablespoons. Creamy salad dressing (such as miracle whip®)
- 5 tablespoons. Mayonnaise
- 25 seedless red grapes, halved

DIRECTIONS

1. In a big bowl, toss together the shredded chicken, lemon juice, apple chunks, celery, red onion, and walnuts.
2. Get another bowl and whisk together the dressing, vanilla yogurt, and mayonnaise. Pour over the chicken mixture. Toss to coat. Fold the grapes carefully into the salad.

NUTRITION: Calories: 307 Total fat: 22.7 g Carbohydrates: 10.8g Protein: 17.3 g Cholesterol: 41 mg Sodium: 128 mg

182. Chicken Strawberry Spinach Salad with Ginger-Lime Dressing

Preparation Time: 10 minutes

Cooking Time: 30 minutes

Servings: 2

INGREDIENTS

- 2 teaspoons. Corn oil
- 1 skinless, boneless chicken breast half - cut into bite-size pieces
- 1/2 teaspoon Garlic powder
- 1 1/2 tablespoons. Mayonnaise
- 1/2 lime, juiced
- 1/2 teaspoon Ground ginger
- 2 teaspoons. Milk
- 2cupfresh spinach, stems removed
- 4 fresh strawberries, sliced
- 1 1/2 tablespoons. Slivered almonds
- Freshly ground black pepper to taste

DIRECTIONS

1. In a skillet, heat oil over medium heat. Add the chicken breast and garlic powder. Cook the chicken for 10 minutes per side. When the juices run clear, remove from heat and set aside.
2. Combine the lime juice, milk, mayonnaise, and ginger in a bowl.
3. Place the spinach on serving dishes. Top with strawberries and chicken. Then sprinkle with almonds. Drizzle the salad with the dressing. Add pepper and serve.

NUTRITION: Calories: 242 Total fat: 17.3 g Carbohydrates: 7.5g Protein: 15.8 g Cholesterol: 40 mg Sodium: 117 mg

183. Asian Chicken Satay

Preparation time: 15 minutes

Cooking time: 10 minutes

Servings: 6

INGREDIENTS

- Juice of 2 limes
- Brown sugar – 2 tablespoons
- Minced garlic – 1 tablespoon
- Ground cumin – 2 teaspoons
- Boneless, skinless chicken breast – 12, cut into strips

DIRECTIONS

1. In a bowl, stir together the cumin, garlic, brown sugar, and lime juice.
2. Add the chicken strips to the bowl and marinate in the refrigerator for 1 hour.
3. Heat the barbecue to medium-high.
4. Remove the chicken from the marinade and thread each strip onto wooden skewers that have been soaked in the water.
5. Grill the chicken for about 4 minutes per side or until the meat is cooked through but still juicy.

NUTRITION: Calories: 78 Carb: 4g Phosphorus: 116mg Potassium: 108mg Sodium: 100mg Protein: 12g

184. Zucchini and Turkey Burger with Jalapeno Peppers

Preparation Time: 15 minutes

Cooking Time: 10 minutes

Servings: 4

INGREDIENTS

- Turkey meat (ground) – 1 pound
- Zucchini (shredded) – 1 cup
- Onion (minced) – ½ cup
- Jalapeño pepper (seeded and minced) – 1
- Egg – 1
- Extra-spicy blend – 1 teaspoon
- Fresh poblano peppers (seeded and sliced in half lengthwise)
- Mustard – 1 teaspoon

DIRECTIONS

1. Start by taking a mixing bowl and adding in the turkey meat, zucchini, onion, jalapeño pepper, egg, and extra-spicy blend. Mix well to combine.
2. Divide the mixture into 4 equal portions. Form burger patties out of the same.
3. Prepare an electric griddle or an outdoor grill. Place the burger patties on the grill and cook until the top is blistered and tender. Place the sliced poblano peppers on the grill alongside the patties. Grilling the patties should take about 5 minutes on each side.
4. Once done, place the patties onto the buns and top them with grilled peppers.

NUTRITION: Protein – 25 g Carbohydrates – 5 g Fat – 10 g Cholesterol – 125 mg Sodium – 128 mg Potassium – 475 mg Phosphorus – 280 mg Calcium – 43 mg Fiber – 1.6 g Name

185. Gnocchi and Chicken Dumplings

Preparation time: 10 minutes

Cooking Time: 40 minutes

Servings: 10

INGREDIENTS

- Chicken breast – 2 pounds
- Gnocchi – 1 pound
- Light olive oil – ¼ cup
- Better Than Bouillon® Chicken Base – 1 tablespoon
- Chicken stock (reduced-sodium) – 6 cups
- Fresh celery (diced finely) – ½ cup
- Fresh onions (diced finely) – ½ cup
- Fresh carrots (diced finely) – ½ cup
- Fresh parsley (chopped) – ¼ cup
- Black pepper – 1 teaspoon
- Italian seasoning – 1 teaspoon

DIRECTIONS

1. Start by placing the stock over a high flame. Add in the oil and let it heat through.
2. Add the chicken to the hot oil and shallow-fry until all sides turn golden brown.
3. Toss in the carrots, onions, and celery and cook for about 5 minutes. Pour in the chicken stock and let it cool on a high flame for about 30 minutes.
4. Reduce the flame and add in the chicken bouillon, Italian seasoning, and black pepper. Stir well.
5. Toss in the store-bought gnocchi and let it cook for about 15 minutes. Keep stirring.
6. Once done, transfer into a serving bowl. Add parsley and serve hot!

NUTRITION: Protein – 28 g Carbohydrates – 38 g Fat – 10 g Cholesterol – 58 mg Sodium – 121 mg Potassium – 485 mg Calcium – 38 mg Fiber – 2 g

MEAT

186. Mouthwatering Beef and Chili Stew

Preparation Time: 15 minutes

Cooking Time: 7 hours

Servings: 6

INGREDIENTS

- 1/2 medium red onion, thinly sliced into half moons
- 1/2 tablespoon vegetable oil
- 10ounce of flat cut beef brisket, whole
- ½ cup low sodium stock
- ¾ cup water
- ½ tablespoon honey
- ½ tablespoon chili powder
- ½ teaspoon smoked paprika
- ½ teaspoon dried thyme
- 1 teaspoon black pepper
- 1 tablespoon corn starch

DIRECTIONS

1. Throw the sliced onion into the slow cooker first.
2. Add a splash of oil to a large hot skillet and briefly seal the beef on all sides.
3. Remove the beef from skillet and place in the slow cooker.
4. Add the stock, water, honey and spices to the same skillet that you cooked the beef in.
5. Loosen the browned bits from bottom of pan with spatula. (Hint: These brown bits at the bottom are called the fond.)
6. Allow juice to simmer until the volume is reduced by about half.
7. Pour the juice over beef in the slow cooker.
8. Set slow cooker on Low and cook for approximately 7 hours.
9. Take the beef out of the slow cooker and onto a platter.
10. Shred it with two forks.
11. Pour the remaining juice into a medium saucepan. Bring to a simmer.
12. Whisk the cornstarch with two tablespoons of water.
13. Add to the juice and cook until slightly thickened.
14. For a thicker sauce, simmer and reduce the juice a bit more before adding cornstarch.
15. Pour the sauce over the meat and serve.

NUTRITION: Per Serving: Calories: 128 Protein: 13g Carbohydrates: 6g Fat: 6g Cholesterol: 39mg Sodium: 228mg Potassium: 202mgPhosphorus: 119mgCalcium: 16mg Fiber: 1g

187. Beef and Three Pepper Stew

Preparation Time: 15 minutes

Cooking Time: 6 hours

Servings: 6

INGREDIENTS

- 10ounce of flat cut beef brisket, whole
- 1 teaspoon of dried thyme
- 1 teaspoon of black pepper
- 1 clove garlic
- ½ cup of green onion, thinly sliced
- ½ cup low sodium chicken stock
- 2 cups water
- 1 large green bell pepper, sliced
- 1 large red bell pepper, sliced
- 1 large yellow bell pepper, sliced
- 1 large red onion, sliced

DIRECTIONS

1. Combine the beef, thyme, pepper, garlic, green onion, stock and water in a slow cooker.
2. Leave it all to cook on High for 4-5 hours until tender.
3. Remove the beef from the slow cooker and let it cool.
4. Shred the beef with two forks and remove any excess fat.
5. Place the shredded beef back into the slow cooker.
6. Add the sliced peppers and the onion.
7. Cook this on High heat for 40-60 minutes until the vegetables are tender.

NUTRITION: Per Serving: Calories: 132 Protein: 14g Carbohydrates: 9g Fat: 5g Cholesterol: 39mg Sodium: 179mg Potassium: 390mg Phosphorus: 141mgCalcium: 33mg Fiber: 2g

188. Sticky Pulled Beef Open Sandwiches

Preparation Time: 15 minutes

Cooking Time: 5 hours

Servings: 5

INGREDIENTS

- ½ cup of green onion, sliced
- 2 garlic cloves
- 2 tablespoons of fresh parsley
- 2 large carrots
- 7ounce of flat cut beef brisket, whole
- 1 tablespoon of smoked paprika
- 1 teaspoon dried parsley
- 1 teaspoon of brown sugar
- ½ teaspoon of black pepper
- 2 tablespoon of olive oil
- ¼ cup of red wine
- 8 tablespoon of cider vinegar
- 3 cups of water
- 5 slices white bread
- 1 cup of arugula to garnish

DIRECTIONS

1. Finely chop the green onion, garlic and fresh parsley.
2. Grate the carrot.
3. Put the beef in to roast in a slow cooker.
4. Add the chopped onion, garlic and remaining ingredients, leaving the rolls, fresh parsley and arugula to one side.
5. Stir in the slow cooker to combine.
6. Cover and cook on Low for 8 1/2 to 10 hours, or on High for 4 to 5 hours until tender. (Hint: Test for tenderness by pressing into the meat with a fork.)
7. Remove the meat from the slow cooker.
8. Shred it apart with two forks.
9. Return the meat to the broth to keep it warm until ready to serve.
10. Lightly toast the bread and top with shredded beef, arugula, fresh parsley and ½ spoon of the broth.
11. Serve.

NUTRITION: Per Serving: Calories: 273 Protein: 15g Carbohydrates: 20g Fat: 11g Cholesterol: 37mg Sodium: 308mg Potassium: 399mg Phosphorus: 159mgCalcium: 113mg Fiber: 3g

189. Herby Beef Stroganoff and Fluffy Rice

Preparation Time: 15 minutes

Cooking Time: 5 hours

Servings: 6

INGREDIENTS

- ½ cup onion
- 2 garlic cloves
- 9ounce of flat cut beef brisket, cut into 1" cubes
- ½ cup of reduced-sodium beef stock
- 1/3 cup red wine
- ½ teaspoon dried oregano
- ¼ teaspoon freshly ground black pepper
- ½ teaspoon dried thyme
- ½ teaspoon of saffron
- ½ cup almond milk (unenriched)
- ¼ cup all-purpose flour
- 1 cup of water
- 2 ½ cups of white rice

DIRECTIONS

1. Chop up the onion and mince the garlic cloves.
2. Mix the beef, stock, wine, onion, garlic, oregano, pepper, thyme and saffron in your slow cooker.
3. Cover and cook on High until the beef is tender, for about 4-5 hours.
4. Combine the almond milk, flour and water.
5. Whisk together until smooth.
6. Add the flour mixture to the slow cooker.
7. Cook for another 15 to 25 minutes until the stroganoff is thick.
8. Cook the rice using the package instructions, leaving out salt.
9. Drain off the excess water.
10. Serve the stroganoff over the rice.

NUTRITION: Per Serving: Calories: 241 Protein: 15g Carbohydrates: 29g Fat: 5g Cholesterol: 39g Sodium: 182mg Potassium: 206mg Phosphorus: 151mgCalcium: 59mg

Meat

191. Chunky Beef and Potato Slow Roast

Preparation Time: 15 minutes

Cooking Time: 5-6 hours

Servings: 12

INGREDIENTS

- 3 cups of peeled potatoes, chunked
- 1 cup of onion
- 2 garlic cloves, chopped
- 1 ¼ pounds flat cut beef brisket, fat trimmed
- 2 of cups water
- 1 teaspoon of chili powder
- 1 tablespoon of dried rosemary

For the sauce:

- 1 tablespoon of freshly grated horseradish
- ½ cup of almond milk (unenriched)
- 1 tablespoon lemon juice (freshly squeezed)
- 1 garlic clove, minced
- A pinch of cayenne pepper

DIRECTIONS

1. Double boil the potatoes to reduce their potassium content.
2. (Hint: Bring your potato to the boil, then drain and refill with water to boil again.)
3. Chop the onion and the garlic.
4. Place the beef brisket in slow cooker.
5. Combine water, chopped garlic, chili powder and rosemary
6. Pour the mixture over the brisket.
7. Cover and cook on High for 4-5 hours until the meat is very tender.
8. Drain the potatoes and add them to the slow cooker.
9. Turn heat to High and cook covered until the potatoes are tender.
10. Prepare the horseradish sauce by whisking together horseradish, milk, lemon juice, minced garlic and cayenne pepper.
11. Cover and refrigerate.
12. Serve your casserole with a dash of horseradish sauce on the side.

NUTRITION: Per Serving: Calories: 199 Protein: 21gCarbohydrates: 12g Fat: 7g Cholesterol: 63mg Sodium: 282mg Potassium: 317 Phosphorus: 191mgCalcium: 23mg Fiber: 1g

192. Spiced Lamb Burgers

Preparation Time: 10 minutes

Cooking Time: 20 minutes

Servings: 2

INGREDIENTS

- 1 tablespoon extra-virgin olive oil
- 1 teaspoon cumin
- ½ finely diced red onion
- 1 minced garlic clove
- 1 teaspoon harissa spices
- 1 cup arugula
- 1 juiced lemon
- 6-ounce lean ground lamb
- 1 tablespoon parsley
- ½ cup low-fat plain yogurt

DIRECTIONS

1. Preheat the broiler on a medium to high heat.
2. Mix together the ground lamb, red onion, parsley, Harissa spices and olive oil until combined.
3. Shape 1-inch thick patties using wet hands.
4. Add the patties to a baking tray and place under the broiler for 7-8 minutes on each side or until thoroughly cooked through.
5. Mix the yogurt, lemon juice and cumin and serve over the lamb burgers with a side salad of arugula.

NUTRITION: Calories 306 Fat 20g Carbs 10g Phosphorus 269mg Potassium (K) 492mg Sodium (Na) 86mg Protein 23g

193. Pork Loins with Leeks

Preparation Time: 10 minutes

Cooking Time: 35 minutes

Servings: 2

INGREDIENTS

- 1 sliced leek
- 1 tablespoon mustard seeds
- 6-ounce Pork tenderloin
- 1 tablespoon cumin seeds
- 1 tablespoon dry mustard
- 1 tablespoon extra-virgin oil

DIRECTIONS

1. Preheat the broiler to medium high heat.
2. In a dry skillet heat mustard and cumin seeds until they start to pop (3-5 minutes).
3. Grind seeds using a pestle and mortar or blender and then mix in the dry mustard.

4. Coat the pork on both sides with the mustard blend and add to a baking tray to broil for 25-30 minutes or until cooked through. Turn once halfway through.
5. Remove and place to one side.
6. Heat the oil in a pan on medium heat and add the leeks for 5-6 minutes or until soft.
7. Serve the pork tenderloin on a bed of leeks and enjoy!

NUTRITION: Calories 139 Fat 5g Carbs 2g Phosphorus 278mg Potassium (K) 45mg Sodium (Na) 47mg Protein 18g

194. Chinese Beef Wraps

Preparation Time: 10 minutes

Cooking Time: 30 minutes

Servings: 2

INGREDIENTS

- 2 iceberg lettuce leaves
- ½ diced cucumber
- 1 teaspoon canola oil
- 5-ounce lean ground beef
- 1 teaspoon ground ginger
- 1 tablespoon chili flakes
- 1 minced garlic clove
- 1 tablespoon rice wine vinegar

DIRECTIONS

1. Mix the ground meat with the garlic, rice wine vinegar, chili flakes and ginger in a bowl.
2. Heat oil in a skillet over medium heat.
3. Add the beef to the pan and cook for 20-25 minutes or until cooked through.
4. Serve beef mixture with diced cucumber in each lettuce wrap and fold.

NUTRITION: Calories 156 Fat 2g Carbs 4 g Phosphorus 1 mg Sodium (Na) 54mg Protein 14g

195. Grilled Skirt Steak

Preparation Time: 15 minutes

Cooking Time: 8-9 minutes

Servings: 4

INGREDIENTS

- 2 teaspoons fresh ginger herb, grated finely
- 2 teaspoons fresh lime zest, grated finely
- ¼ cup coconut sugar
- 2 teaspoons fish sauce
- 2 tablespoons fresh lime juice
- ½ cup coconut milk
- 1-pound beef skirt steak, trimmed and cut into 4-inch slices lengthwise

- Salt, to taste

DIRECTIONS

1. In a sizable sealable bag, mix together all ingredients except steak and salt.
2. Add steak and coat with marinade generously.
3. Seal the bag and refrigerate to marinate for about 4-12 hours.
4. Preheat the grill to high heat. Grease the grill grate.
5. Remove steak from refrigerator and discard the marinade.
6. With a paper towel, dry the steak and sprinkle with salt evenly.
7. Cook the steak for approximately 3½ minutes.
8. Flip the medial side and cook for around 2½-5 minutes or till desired doneness.
9. Remove from grill pan and keep side for approximately 5 minutes before slicing.
10. With a clear, crisp knife cut into desired slices and serve.

NUTRITION: Calories: 465 Fat: 10g Carbohydrates: 22g Fiber: 0g Protein: 37g

196. Spicy Lamb Curry

Preparation Time: 15 minutes

Cooking Time: 2 hours 15 minutes

Servings: 6-8

INGREDIENTS

- 4 teaspoons ground coriander
- 4 teaspoons ground coriander
- 4 teaspoons ground cumin
- ¾ teaspoon ground ginger
- 2 teaspoons ground cinnamon
- ½ teaspoon ground cloves
- ½ teaspoon ground cardamom
- 2 tablespoons sweet paprika
- ½ tablespoon cayenne pepper
- 2 teaspoons chili powder
- 2 teaspoons salt
- 1 tablespoon coconut oil
- 2 pounds boneless lamb, trimmed and cubed into 1-inch size
- Salt and freshly ground black pepper, to taste
- 2 cups onions, chopped
- 1¼ cups water
- 1 cup coconut milk

DIRECTIONS

1. For spice mixture in a bowl, mix together all spices. Keep aside.
2. Season the lamb with salt and black pepper.

3. In a large Dutch oven, heat oil on medium-high heat.
4. Add lamb and stir fry for around 5 minutes.
5. Add onion and cook approximately 4-5 minutes.
6. Stir in spice mixture and cook approximately 1 minute.
7. Add water and coconut milk and provide to some boil on high heat.
8. Reduce the heat to low and simmer, covered for approximately 1-120 minutes or till desired doneness of lamb.
9. Uncover and simmer for approximately 3-4 minutes.
10. Serve hot.

NUTRITION: Calories: 466 Fat: 10g Carbohydrates: 23g Fiber: 9g Protein: 36g

197. Lamb with Prunes

Preparation Time: 15 minutes

Cooking Time: 2 hours and 40 minutes

Servings: 4-6

INGREDIENTS

- 3 tablespoons coconut oil
- 2 onions, chopped finely
- 1 (1-inch) piece fresh ginger, minced
- 3 garlic cloves, minced
- ½ teaspoon ground turmeric
- 2 ½ pound lamb shoulder, trimmed and cubed into 3-inch size
- Salt and freshly ground black pepper, to taste
- ½ teaspoon saffron threads, crumbled
- 1 cinnamon stick
- 3 cups water
- 1 cup runes, pitted and halved

DIRECTIONS

1. In a big pan, melt coconut oil on medium heat.
2. Add onions, ginger, garlic cloves and turmeric and sauté for about 3-5 minutes.
3. Sprinkle the lamb with salt and black pepper evenly.
4. In the pan, add lamb and saffron threads and cook for approximately 4-5 minutes.
5. Add cinnamon stick and water and produce to some boil on high heat.
6. Reduce the temperature to low and simmer, covered for around 1½-120 minutes or till desired doneness of lamb.
7. Stir in prunes and simmer for approximately 20-a half-hour.
8. Remove cinnamon stick and serve hot.

NUTRITION: Calories: 393 Fat: 12g Carbohydrates: 10g Fiber: 4g Protein: 36g

198. Roast Beef

Preparation Time: 25 minutes

Cooking Time: 55 minutes

Servings: 3

INGREDIENTS

- Quality rump or sirloin tip roast
- Direction:
- Place in roasting pan o n a shallow rack
- Season with pepper and herbs
- Insert meat thermometer in the center or thickest part of the roast
- Roast to the desired degree of doneness
- After removing from over for about 15 minutes let it chill
- In the end the roast should be moister than well done.

NUTRITION: Calories 158 Protein 24 g Fat 6 g Carbs 0 g Phosphorus 206 mg Potassium (K) 328 mg Sodium (Na) 55 mg

199. Beef Brochettes

Preparation Time: 20 minutes

Cooking Time: 1 hour

Servings: 1

INGREDIENTS

- 1 ½ cups pineapple chunks
- 1 sliced large onion
- 2 pounds thick steak
- 1 sliced medium bell pepper
- 1 bay leaf
- ¼ cup vegetable oil
- ½ cup lemon juice
- 2 crushed garlic cloves

DIRECTIONS

1. Cut beef cubes and place in a plastic bag
2. Combine marinade ingredients in small bowl
3. Mix and pour over beef cubes
4. Seal the bag and refrigerate for 3 to 5 hours
5. Divide ingredients onion, beef cube, green pepper, pineapple
6. Grill about 9 minutes each side

NUTRITION: Calories 304 Protein 35 g Fat 15 g Carbs 11 g Phosphorus 264 mg Potassium (K) 388 mg Sodium (Na) 70 mg

200. Country Fried Steak

Preparation Time: 10 minutes

Cooking Time: 1 hour and 40 minutes

Servings: 3

INGREDIENTS

- 1 large onion
- ½ cup flour
- 3 tablespoons. vegetable oil
- ¼ teaspoon pepper
- 1½ pounds round steak
- ½ teaspoon paprika

DIRECTIONS

1. Trim excess fat from steak
2. Cut into small pieces
3. Combine flour, paprika and pepper and mix together
4. Preheat skillet with oil
5. Cook steak on both sides
6. When the color of steak is brown remove to a platter
7. Add water (150 ml) and stir around the skillet
8. Return browned steak to skillet, if necessary, add water again so that bottom side of steak does not stick

NUTRITION: Calories 248 Protein 30 g Fat 10 g Carbs 5 g Phosphorus 190 mg Potassium (K) 338 mg Sodium (Na) 60 mg

201. Beef Pot Roast

Preparation Time: 20 minutes

Cooking Time: 1 hour

Servings: 3

INGREDIENTS

- Round bone roast
- 2 - 4 pounds chuck roast
- Direction:
- Trim off excess fat
- Place a tablespoon of oil in a large skillet and heat to medium
- Roll pot roast in flour and brown on all sides in a hot skillet
- After the meat gets a brown color, reduce heat to low
- Season with pepper and herbs and add ½ cup of water
- Cook slowly for 1½ hours or until it looks ready

NUTRITION: Calories 157 Protein 24 g Fat 13 g Carbs 0 g Phosphorus 204 mg Sodium (Na) 50 mg

202. Homemade Burgers

Preparation Time: 10 minutes

Cooking Time: 20 minutes

Servings: 2

INGREDIENTS

- 4 ounce lean 100% ground beef
- 1 teaspoon black pepper
- 1 garlic clove, minced
- 1 teaspoon olive oil
- 1/4 cup onion, finely diced
- 1 tablespoon balsamic vinegar
- 1/2ounce brie cheese, crumbled
- 1 teaspoon mustard

DIRECTIONS

1. Season ground beef with pepper and then mix in minced garlic.
2. Form burger shapes with the ground beef using the palms of your hands.
3. Heat a skillet on a medium to high heat, and then add the oil.
4. Sauté the onions for 5-10 minutes until browned.
5. Then add the balsamic vinegar and sauté for another 5 minutes.
6. Remove and set aside.
7. Add the burgers to the pan and heat on the same heat for 5-6 minutes before flipping and heating for a further 5-6 minutes until cooked through.
8. Spread the mustard onto each burger.
9. Crumble the brie cheese over each burger and serve!
10. Try with a crunchy side salad!
11. Tip: If using fresh beef and not defrosted, prepare double the ingredients and freeze burgers in plastic wrap (after cooling) for up to 1 month.
12. Thoroughly defrost before heating through completely in the oven to serve.

NUTRITION: Calories: 178 Fat: 10g Carbohydrates: 4g Phosphorus: 147mg Potassium: 272mg Sodium: 273 mg Protein: 16g

203. Slow-cooked Beef Brisket

Preparation Time: 10 minutes

Cooking Time: 3 hours and 30 minutes

Servings: 6

INGREDIENTS

- 10-ounce chuck roast
- 1 onion, sliced
- 1 cup carrots, peeled and sliced
- 1 tablespoon mustard
- 1 tablespoon thyme (fresh or dried)
- 1 tablespoon rosemary (fresh or dried)
- 2 garlic cloves
- 2 tablespoon extra-virgin olive oil
- 1 teaspoon black pepper
- 1 cup homemade chicken stock (p.52)
- 1 cup water

DIRECTIONS

1. Preheat oven to 300°f/150°c/Gas Mark 2.
2. Trim any fat from the beef and soak vegetables in warm water.
3. Make a paste by mixing together the mustard, thyme, rosemary, and garlic, before mixing in the oil and pepper.
4. Combine this mix with the stock.
5. Pour the mixture over the beef into an oven proof baking dish.
6. Place the vegetables onto the bottom of the baking dish with the beef.
7. Cover and roast for 3 hours, or until tender.
8. Uncover the dish and continue to cook for 30 minutes in the oven.
9. Serve hot!

NUTRITION: Calories: 151 Fat: 7g Carbohydrates: 7g Phosphorus: 144mg Potassium: 344mg Sodium: 279mg Protein: 15g

204. Pork Souvlaki

Preparation time: 20 minutes

Cooking time: 12 minutes

Servings: 8

INGREDIENTS

- Olive oil – 3 tablespoons
- Lemon juice – 2 tablespoons
- Minced garlic – 1 teaspoon
- Chopped fresh oregano – 1 tablespoon
- Ground black pepper – ¼ teaspoon
- Pork leg – 1 pound, cut in 2-inch cubes

DIRECTIONS

1. In a bowl, stir together the lemon juice, olive oil, garlic, oregano, and pepper.
2. Add the pork cubes and toss to coat.
3. Place the bowl in the refrigerator, covered, for 2 hours to marinate.
4. Thread the pork chunks onto 8 wooden skewers that have been soaked in water.
5. Preheat the barbecue to medium-high heat.
6. Grill the pork skewers for about 12 minutes, turning once, until just cooked through but still juicy.

NUTRITION: Calories: 95 Fat: 4g Carb: 0g Phosphorus: 125mg Potassium: 230mg Sodium: 29mg Protein: 13g

205. Open-Faced Beef Stir-Up

Preparation time: 10 minutes

Cooking time: 10 minutes

Servings: 6

INGREDIENTS

- 95% Lean ground beef – ½ pound
- Chopped sweet onion – ½ cup
- Shredded cabbage – ½ cup
- Herb pesto – ¼ cup
- Hamburger buns – 6, bottom halves only

DIRECTIONS

1. Sauté the beef and onion for 6 minutes or until beef is cooked.
2. Add the cabbage and sauté for 3 minutes more.
3. Stir in pesto and heat for 1 minute.
4. Divide the beef mixture into 6 portions and serve each on the bottom half of a hamburger bun, open-face.

NUTRITION: Calories: 120 Fat: 3g Phosphorus: 106mg Potassium: 198mg Sodium: 134mg Protein: 11g

206. Grilled Steak with Cucumber Salsa

Preparation time: 20 minutes

Cooking time: 15 minutes

Servings: 4

INGREDIENTS

For the salsa

- Chopped English cucumber - 1 cup
- Boiled and diced red bell pepper – ¼ cup
- Scallion – 1, both green and white parts, chopped
- Chopped fresh cilantro – 2 tablespoons
- Juice of 1 lime

For the steak
- Beef tenderloin steaks – 4 (3-ounce), room temperature
- Olive oil
- Freshly ground black pepper

DIRECTIONS
1. To make the salsa, in a bowl combine the lime juice, cilantro, scallion, bell pepper, and cucumber. Set aside.
2. To make the steak: Preheat a barbecue to medium heat.
3. Rub the steaks all over with oil and season with pepper.
4. Grill the steaks for about 5 minutes per side for medium-rare, or until the desired state.
5. Serve the steaks topped with salsa.

NUTRITION: Calories: 130 Fat: 6g Carb: 1g Phosphorus: 186mg Potassium: 272mg Sodium: 39mg Protein: 19g

207. Beef Brisket

Preparation time: 10 minutes

Cooking time: 3 ½ hours

Servings: 6

INGREDIENTS
- Chuck roast – 12 ounces trimmed
- Garlic – 2 cloves
- Thyme – 1 tablespoon
- Rosemary – tablespoon
- Mustard - 1 tablespoon
- Extra virgin olive oil – ¼ cup
- Black pepper – 1 teaspoon
- Onion – 1, diced
- Carrots – 1 cup, peeled and sliced
- Low salt stock – 2 cups

DIRECTIONS
1. Preheat the oven to 300F.
2. Soak vegetables in warm water.
3. Make a paste by mixing together the thyme, mustard, rosemary, and garlic. Then mix in the oil and pepper.
4. Add the beef to the dish.
5. Pour the mixture over the beef into a dish.
6. Place the vegetables onto the bottom of the baking dish around the beef.
7. Cover and roast for 3 hours, or until tender.
8. Uncover the dish and continue to cook for 30 minutes in the oven.
9. Serve.

NUTRITION: Calories: 303 Fat: 25g Carb: 7g Phosphorus: 376mg Potassium: 246mg Sodium: 44mg Protein: 18g

208. Apricot and Lamb Tagine

Preparation time: 10 minutes

Cooking time: 1 to 1 ½ hours

Servings: 2

INGREDIENTS
- Extra virgin olive oil – 1 tablespoon
- Lean lamb fillets – 2, cubed
- Onion – 1, diced
- Homemade chicken stock – 4 cups
- Cumin – 1 teaspoon
- Turmeric – 1 teaspoon
- Curry powder – 1 teaspoon
- Dried rosemary – 1 teaspoon
- Chopped parsley – 1 teaspoon
- Canned apricots – ½ cup, juices drained and apricots rinsed

DIRECTIONS
1. Heat the olive oil in a pot.
2. Add lamb to the pot and cook for 5 minutes or until browned.
3. Remove lamb and set aside.
4. Add the chopped onion to the pot and sauté for 5 minutes, or until starting to soften.
5. Sprinkle with cumin, curry powder, and turmeric over the onions and continue to stir for 4 to 5 minutes.
6. Now add the lamb back into the pot with the chicken stock and rosemary.
7. Cover the pot and leave to simmer on a low heat for 1 to 1.5 hours or until the lamb is tender and fully cooked through.
8. Add the apricots 15 minutes before the end of the cooking time.
9. Garnish with parsley and serve.

NUTRITION: Calories: 193 Fat: 12g Carb: 9g Phosphorus: 170mg Potassium: 156mg Sodium: 105mg Protein: 20g

209. Lamb Shoulder with Zucchini and Eggplant

Preparation time: 10 minutes

Cooking time: 4 to 5 hours

Servings: 2

INGREDIENTS

- Lean lamb shoulder – 6 ounces
- Zucchinis – 2, cubed
- Eggplant – 1, cubed
- Black pepper – 1 teaspoon
- Extra virgin olive oil – 2 tablespoons
- Basil – 1 tablespoon
- Oregano – 1 tablespoon
- Garlic – 2 cloves, chopped

DIRECTIONS

1. Preheat the oven to its highest setting.
2. Soak the vegetables in warm water.
3. Trim any fat from the lamb shoulder.
4. Rub the lamb with 1 tablespoon olive oil, pepper, and herbs.
5. Line a baking tray with the rest of the olive oil, garlic, zucchini, and eggplant.
6. Add the lamb shoulder and cover with foil.
7. Turn the oven down to 325F and add the dish into the oven.
8. Cook for 4 to 5 hours, remove and rest.
9. Slice the lamb and then serve with the vegetables.

NUTRITION: Calories: 478 Fat: 31g Carb: 13g Phosphorus: 197mg Potassium: 414mg Sodium: 84mg Protein: 33g

210. Beef Chili

Preparation time: 10 minutes

Cooking time: 30 minutes

Servings: 2

INGREDIENTS

- Onion – 1, diced
- Red bell pepper – 1, diced
- Garlic – 2 cloves, minced
- Lean ground beef – 6 ounces
- Chili powder – 1 teaspoon
- Oregano – 1 teaspoon
- Extra virgin olive oil – 2 tablespoons
- Water – 1 cup
- Brown rice -1 cup
- Fresh cilantro – 1 tablespoon, to serve

DIRECTIONS

1. Soak vegetables in warm water.
2. Bring a pan of water to the boil and add rice for 20 minutes.
3. Meanwhile, add the oil to a pan and heat on medium-high heat.
4. Add the pepper, onions, and garlic and sauté for 5 minutes until soft.
5. Remove and set aside.
6. Add the beef to the pan and stir until browned.
7. Add the vegetables back into the pan and stir.
8. Now add the chili powder and herbs and water, cover and turn the heat down a little to simmer for 15 minutes.
9. Meanwhile, drain the water from the rice, add the lid and steam while the chili is cooking.
10. Serve hot with the fresh cilantro sprinkled over the top.

NUTRITION: Calories: 459 Fat: 22g Carb: 36g Phosphorus: 332mg Potassium: 360mg Protein: 22g

211. Skirt Steak Glazed with Bourbon

Preparation Time: 30 minutes

Cooking Time: 50 minutes (1 hour additional)

Servings: 8

INGREDIENTS

- Bourbon Glaze
- Shallots (diced) – ¼ cup
- Unsalted butter (chilled) – 3 tablespoons
- Bourbon – 1 cup
- Dark brown sugar – ¼ cup
- Dijon mustard – 2 tablespoons
- Black pepper – 1 tablespoon
- Skirt Steak
- Grapeseed oil – 2 tablespoons
- Dried oregano – ½ teaspoon
- Smoked paprika – ½ teaspoon
- Black pepper – 1 teaspoon
- Red wine vinegar – 1 tablespoon
- Skirt steak – 2 pounds

DIRECTIONS

1. Start by preparing the bourbon glaze. For this, you will need to take a small saucepan and place it over a medium-high flame.
2. Add in 1 tablespoon of butter and toss in the shallots. Stir-fry until they turn brown.
3. Reduce the heat to the minimum and remove the saucepan from the stove. Pour in the bourbon and stir thoroughly. Return the saucepan to the stove.
4. Let this cook on a low flame for about 15 minutes. Make sure the glaze reduces to one-third.

5. Stir in the dark sugar, black pepper, and Dijon mustard. Keep stirring until the glaze becomes bubbly.
6. Turn off the flame and add in about 2 tablespoons of cold butter. Keep stirring to incorporate with the sauce.
7. Now prepare the skirt steak. To do this, take a gallon-sized zip-lock bag and add in the grapeseed oil, dried oregano, smoked paprika, black pepper, and red wine vinegar. Mix well.
8. Now add in the steaks and shake well. Allow the steaks to sit in the marinade for about 45 minutes.
9. Remove the steaks from the zip-lock bag. Set aside.
10. Heat the grill and place the steaks on it. Cook for about 20 minutes.
11. Once done, remove the steak and place it on a baking tray. Let it rest for about 10 minutes before serving.
12. Slice the steaks and drizzle the glaze on top. Place the tray in the broiler for 5 minutes. Serve hot!

NUTRITION: Protein – 24 g Carbohydrates – 8 g Fat – 22 g Cholesterol – 93 mg Sodium – 152 mg Potassium – 283 mg Phosphorus – 171 mg Calcium – 22 mg Fiber – 0.5 g

DESSERTS

212. Dessert Cocktail

Preparation Time: 1 minutes

Cooking Time: 0 minute

Servings: 4

INGREDIENTS

- 1 cup of cranberry juice
- 1 cup of fresh ripe strawberries, washed and hull removed
- 2 tablespoon of lime juice
- ¼ cup of white sugar
- 8 ice cubes

DIRECTIONS

1. Combine all the ingredients in a blender until smooth and creamy.
2. Pour the liquid into chilled tall glasses and serve cold.

NUTRITION: Calories: 92 kcal Carbohydrate: 23.5 g Protein: 0.5 g Sodium: 3.62 mg Potassium: 103.78 mg Phosphorus: 17.86 mg Dietary Fiber: 0.84 g Fat: 0.17 g

213. Baked Egg Custard

Preparation Time: 15 minutes

Cooking Time: 30 minutes

Servings: 4

INGREDIENTS

- 2 medium eggs, at room temperature
- ¼ cup of semi-skimmed milk
- 3 tablespoons of white sugar
- ½ teaspoon of nutmeg
- 1 teaspoon of vanilla extract

DIRECTIONS

1. Preheat your oven at 375 F/180C
2. Mix all the ingredients in a mixing bowl and beat with a hand mixer for a few seconds until creamy and uniform.
3. Pour the mixture into lightly greased muffin tins.
4. Bake for 25-30 minutes or until the knife, you place inside, comes out clean.

NUTRITION: Calories: 96.56 kcal Carbohydrate: 10.5 g Protein: 3.5 g Sodium: 37.75 mg Potassium: 58.19 mg Phosphorus: 58.76 mg Dietary Fiber: 0.06 g Fat: 2.91 g

214. Gumdrop Cookies

Preparation Time: 15 minutes

Cooking Time: 12 minutes

Servings: 25

INGREDIENTS

- ½ cup of spreadable unsalted butter
- 1 medium egg
- 1 cup of brown sugar
- 1 ⅔ cups of all-purpose flour, sifted
- ¼ cup of milk
- 1 teaspoon vanilla
- 1 teaspoon of baking powder
- 15 large gumdrops, chopped finely

DIRECTIONS

1. Preheat the oven at 400F/195C.
2. Combine the sugar, butter and egg until creamy.
3. Add the milk and vanilla and stir well.
4. Combine the flour with the baking powder in a different bowl. Incorporate to the sugar, butter mixture, and stir.
5. Add the gumdrops and place the mixture in the fridge for half an hour.
6. Drop the dough with tablespoonful into a lightly greased baking or cookie sheet.
7. Bake for 10-12 minutes or until golden brown in color.

NUTRITION: Calories: 102.17 kcal Carbohydrate: 16.5 g Protein: 0.86 g Sodium: 23.42 mg Potassium: 45 mg Phosphorus: 32.15 mg Dietary Fiber: 0.13 g Fat: 4 g

215. Pound Cake with Pineapple

Preparation Time: 10 minutes

Cooking Time: 50 minutes

Servings: 24

INGREDIENTS

- 3 cups of all-purpose flour, sifted
- 3 cups of sugar
- 1 ½ cups of butter
- 6 whole eggs and 3 egg whites
- 1 teaspoon of vanilla extract
- 1 10. ounce can of pineapple chunks, rinsed and crushed (keep juice aside).

For glaze:

- 1 cup of sugar
- 1 stick of unsalted butter or margarine
- Reserved juice from the pineapple

DIRECTIONS

1. Preheat the oven at 350F/180C.

2. Beat the sugar and the butter with a hand mixer until creamy and smooth.
3. Slowly add the eggs (one or two every time) and stir well after pouring each egg.
4. Add the vanilla extract, follow up with the flour and stir well.
5. Add the drained and chopped pineapple.
6. Pour the mixture into a greased cake tin and bake for 45-50 minutes.
7. In a small saucepan, combine the sugar with the butter and pineapple juice. Stir every few seconds and bring to boil. Cook until you get a creamy to thick glaze consistency.
8. Pour the glaze over the cake while still hot.
9. Let cook for at least 10 seconds and serve.

NUTRITION: Calories: 407.4 kcal Carbohydrate: 79 g Protein: 4.25 g Sodium: 118.97 mg Potassium: 180.32 mg Phosphorus: 66.37 mg Dietary Fiber: 2.25 g Fat: 16.48 g

216. Apple Crunch Pie

Preparation Time: 10 minutes

Cooking Time: 35 minutes

Servings: 8

INGREDIENTS

- 4 large tart apples, peeled, seeded and sliced
- ½ cup of white all-purpose flour
- ⅓ cup margarine
- 1 cup of sugar
- ¾ cup of rolled oat flakes
- ½ teaspoon of ground nutmeg

DIRECTIONS

1. Preheat the oven to 375F/180C.
2. Place the apples over a lightly greased square pan (around 7 inches).
3. Mix the rest of the ingredients in a medium bowl with and spread the batter over the apples.
4. Bake for 30-35 minutes or until the top crust has gotten golden brown.
5. Serve hot.

NUTRITION: Calories: 261.9 kcal Carbohydrate: 47.2 g Protein: 1.5 g Sodium: 81 mg Potassium: 123.74 mg Phosphorus: 35.27 mg Dietary Fiber: 2.81 g Fat: 7.99 g

217. Spiced Peaches

Preparation Time: 5 minutes

Cooking Time: 10 minutes

Servings: 2

INGREDIENTS

- Canned peaches with juices – 1 cup
- Cornstarch – ½ teaspoon
- Ground cloves – 1 teaspoon
- Ground cinnamon – 1 teaspoon
- Ground nutmeg – 1 teaspoon
- Zest of ½ lemon
- Water – ½ cup

DIRECTIONS

1. Drain peaches.
2. Combine cinnamon, cornstarch, nutmeg, ground cloves, and lemon zest in a pan on the stove.
3. Heat on a medium heat and add peaches.
4. Bring to a boil, reduce the heat and simmer for 10 minutes.
5. Serve.

NUTRITION: Calories: 70 Fat: 0g Carb: 14g Phosphorus: 23mg Potassium: 176mg Sodium: 3mg Protein: 1g

218. Pumpkin Cheesecake Bar

Preparation Time: 10 minutes

Cooking Time: 50 minutes

Servings: 4

INGREDIENTS

- Unsalted butter – 2 ½ Tablespoons.
- Cream cheese – 4 ounces
- All-purpose white flour – ½ cup
- Golden brown sugar – 3 Tablespoons.
- Granulated sugar – ¼ cup
- Pureed pumpkin – ½ cup
- Egg whites - 2
- Ground cinnamon – 1 teaspoon
- Ground nutmeg – 1 teaspoon
- Vanilla extract – 1 teaspoon

DIRECTIONS

1. Preheat the oven to 350F.
2. Mix flour and brown sugar in a bowl.
3. Mix in the butter to form 'breadcrumbs.
4. Place ¾ of this mixture in a dish.
5. Bake in the oven for 15 minutes. Remove and cool.
6. Lightly whisk the egg and fold in the cream cheese, sugar, pumpkin, cinnamon, nutmeg and vanilla until smooth.
7. Pour this mixture over the oven-baked base and sprinkle with the rest of the breadcrumbs from earlier.
8. Bake in the oven for 30 to 35 minutes more.
9. Cool, slice and serve.

NUTRITION: Calories: 248 Fat: 13g Carb: 33g Phosphorus: 67mg Potassium: 96mg Sodium: 146mg Protein: 4g

Desserts

219. Blueberry Mini Muffins

Preparation Time: 10 minutes

Cooking Time: 35 minutes

Servings: 4

INGREDIENTS

- Egg whites – 3
- All-purpose white flour – ¼ cup
- Coconut flour – 1 Tablespoon
- Baking soda – 1 teaspoon
- Nutmeg – 1 Tablespoon grated
- Vanilla extract – 1 teaspoon
- Stevia – 1 teaspoon
- Fresh blueberries – ¼ cup

DIRECTIONS

1. Preheat the oven to 325F.
2. Mix all the ingredients in a bowl.
3. Divide the batter into 4 and spoon into a lightly oiled muffin tin.
4. Bake in the oven for 15 to 20 minutes or until cooked through.
5. Cool and serve.

NUTRITION: Calories: 62 Fat: 0g Carb: 9g Phosphorus: 103mg Potassium: 65mg Sodium: 62mg Protein: 4g

220. Vanilla Custard

Preparation Time: 7 minutes

Cooking Time: 10 minutes

Servings: 10

INGREDIENTS

- Egg – 1
- Vanilla – 1/8 teaspoon
- Nutmeg – 1/8 teaspoon
- Almond milk – ½ cup
- Stevia - 2 Tablespoon

DIRECTIONS

1. Scald the milk then let it cool slightly.
2. Break the egg into a bowl and beat it with the nutmeg.
3. Add the scalded milk, the vanilla, and the sweetener to taste. Mix well.
4. Place the bowl in a baking pan filled with ½ deep of water.
5. Bake for 30 minutes at 325F.
6. Serve.

NUTRITION: Calories: 167.3 Fat: 9g Carb: 11g Phosphorus: 205mg Potassium: 249mg Sodium: 124mg Protein: 10g

221. Chocolate Chip Cookies

Preparation Time: 7 minutes

Cooking Time: 10 minutes

Servings: 10

INGREDIENTS

- Semi-sweet chocolate chips – ½ cup
- Baking soda – ½ teaspoon
- Vanilla – ½ teaspoon
- Egg – 1
- Flour – 1 cup
- Margarine – ½ cup
- Stevia – 4 teaspoons

DIRECTIONS

1. Sift the dry ingredients.
2. Cream the margarine, stevia, vanilla and egg with a whisk.
3. Add flour mixture and beat well.
4. Stir in the chocolate chips, then drop teaspoonfuls of the mixture over a greased baking sheet.
5. Bake the cookies for about 10 minutes at 375F.
6. Cool and serve.

NUTRITION: Calories: 106.2 Fat: 7g Carb: 8.9g Phosphorus: 19mg Potassium: 28mg Sodium: 98mg Protein: 1.5g

222. Lemon Mousse

Preparation Time: 10 + chill time

Cooking Time: 10 minutes

Servings: 4

INGREDIENTS

- 1 cup coconut cream
- 8 ounces cream cheese, soft
- ¼ cup fresh lemon juice
- 3 pinches salt
- 1 teaspoon lemon liquid stevia

DIRECTIONS

1. Preheat your oven to 350 °F
2. Grease a ramekin with butter
3. Beat cream, cream cheese, fresh lemon juice, salt and lemon liquid stevia in a mixer
4. Pour batter into ramekin
5. Bake for 10 minutes, then transfer the mousse to a serving glass
6. Let it chill for 2 hours and serve
7. Enjoy!

NUTRITION: Calories: 395 Fat: 31g Carbohydrates: 3g Protein: 5g

223. Jalapeno Crisp

Preparation Time: 10 minutes

Cooking Time: 1 hour 15 minutes

Servings: 20

INGREDIENTS

- 1 cup sesame seeds
- 1 cup sunflower seeds
- 1 cup flaxseeds
- ½ cup hulled hemp seeds
- 3 tablespoons Psyllium husk
- 1 teaspoon salt
- 1 teaspoon baking powder
- 2 cups of water

DIRECTIONS

1. Pre-heat your oven to 350 °F
2. Take your blender and add seeds, baking powder, salt, and Psyllium husk
3. Blend well until a sand-like texture appears
4. Stir in water and mix until a batter form
5. Allow the batter to rest for 10 minutes until a dough-like thick mixture forms
6. Pour the dough onto a cookie sheet lined with parchment paper
7. Spread it evenly, making sure that it has a thickness of ¼ inch thick all around
8. Bake for 75 minutes in your oven
9. Remove and cut into 20 spices
10. Allow them to cool for 30 minutes and enjoy!

NUTRITION: Calories: 156 Fat: 13g Carbohydrates: 2g Protein: 5g

224. Raspberry Popsicle

Preparation Time: 2 hours

Cooking Time: 15 minutes

Servings: 4

INGREDIENTS

- 1 ½ cups raspberries
- 2 cups of water

DIRECTIONS

1. Take a pan and fill it up with water
2. Add raspberries
3. Place it over medium heat and bring to water to a boil
4. Reduce the heat and simmer for 15 minutes
5. Remove heat and pour the mix into Popsicle molds
6. Add a popsicle stick and let it chill for 2 hours
7. Serve and enjoy!

NUTRITION: Calories: 58 Fat: 0.4g Carbohydrates: 0g Protein: 1.4g

225. Easy Fudge

Preparation Time: 15 minutes + chill time

Cooking Time: 5 minutes

Servings: 25

INGREDIENTS

- 1 ¾ cups of coconut butter
- 1 cup pumpkin puree
- 1 teaspoon ground cinnamon
- ¼ teaspoon ground nutmeg
- 1 tablespoon coconut oil

DIRECTIONS

1. Take an 8x8 inch square baking pan and line it with aluminum foil
2. Take a spoon and scoop out the coconut butter into a heated pan and allow the butter to melt
3. Keep stirring well and remove from the heat once fully melted
4. Add spices and pumpkin and keep straining until you have a grain-like texture
5. Add coconut oil and keep stirring to incorporate everything
6. Scoop the mixture into your baking pan and evenly distribute it
7. Place wax paper on top of the mixture and press gently to straighten the top
8. Remove the paper and discard
9. Allow it to chill for 1-2 hours
10. Once chilled, take it out and slice it up into pieces
11. Enjoy!

NUTRITION: Calories: 120 Fat: 10g Carbohydrates: 5g Protein: 1.2g

226. Coconut Loaf

Preparation Time: 15 minutes

Cooking Time: 40 minutes

Servings: 4

INGREDIENTS

- 1 ½ tablespoons coconut flour
- ¼ teaspoon baking powder
- 1/8 teaspoon salt
- 1 tablespoon coconut oil, melted
- 1 whole egg

DIRECTIONS

1. Preheat your oven to 350 °F
2. Add coconut flour, baking powder, salt
3. Add coconut oil, eggs and stir well until mixed

Desserts

4. Leave the batter for several minutes
5. Pour half the batter onto the baking pan
6. Spread it to form a circle, repeat with remaining batter
7. Bake in the oven for 10 minutes
8. Once a golden-brown texture comes, let it cool and serve
9. Enjoy!

NUTRITION: Calories: 297 Fat: 14g Carbohydrates: 15g Protein: 15g

227. Chocolate Parfait

Preparation Time: 2 hours

Cooking Time: 0 minute

Servings: 4

INGREDIENTS

- Take a bowl and add cocoa powder, almond milk, chia seeds, vanilla extract, and stir
- Transfer to dessert glass and place in your fridge for 2 hours
- Serve and enjoy!

DIRECTIONS

1. Take a bowl and add cocoa powder, almond milk, chia seeds, vanilla extract, and stir
2. Transfer to dessert glass and place in your fridge for 2 hours
3. Serve and enjoy!

NUTRITION: Calories: 130 Fat: 5g Carbohydrates: 7g Protein: 16g

228. Cauliflower Bagel

Preparation Time: 10 minutes

Cooking Time: 30 minutes

Servings: 12

INGREDIENTS

- 1 large cauliflower, divided into florets and roughly chopped
- ¼ cup nutritional yeast
- ¼ cup almond flour
- ½ teaspoon garlic powder
- 1 ½ teaspoon fine sea salt
- 2 whole eggs
- 1 tablespoon sesame seeds

DIRECTIONS

1. Preheat your oven to 400 °F
2. Line a baking sheet with parchment paper, keep it on the side
3. Blend cauliflower in a food processor and transfer to a bowl

4. Add nutritional yeast, almond flour, garlic powder and salt to a bowl, mix
5. Take another bowl and whisk in eggs, add to cauliflower mix
6. Give the dough a stir
7. Incorporate the mix into the egg mix
8. Make balls from the dough, making a hole using your thumb into each ball
9. Arrange them on your prepped sheet, flattening them into bagel shapes
10. Sprinkle sesame seeds and bake for half an hour
11. Remove the oven and let them cool, enjoy!

NUTRITION: Calories: 152 Fat: 10g Carbohydrates: 4g Protein: 4g

229. Almond Crackers

Preparation Time: 10 minutes

Cooking Time: 20 minutes

Servings: 40 crackers

INGREDIENTS

- 1 cup almond flour
- ¼ teaspoon baking soda
- ¼ teaspoon salt
- 1/8 teaspoon black pepper
- 3 tablespoons sesame seeds
- 1 egg, beaten
- Salt and pepper to taste

DIRECTIONS

1. Preheat your oven to 350 °F
2. Line two baking sheets with parchment paper and keep them on the side
3. Mix the dry ingredients into a large bowl and add egg, mix well and form a dough
4. Divide dough into two balls
5. Roll out the dough. Do this between two pieces of parchment paper.
6. Cut into crackers and transfer them to prep a baking sheet
7. Bake for 15-20 minutes
8. Repeat this process until all the dough has been used up
9. Leave crackers to cool and serve
10. Enjoy!

NUTRITION: Calories: 302 Fat: 28g Carbohydrates: 4g Protein: 9g

230. Cashew and Almond Butter

Preparation Time: 5 minutes

Cooking Time: 15 minutes

Servings: 1 ½ cups

INGREDIENTS

- 1 cup almonds, blanched
- 1/3 cup cashew nuts
- 2 tablespoons coconut oil
- Salt as needed
- ½ teaspoon cinnamon

DIRECTIONS

1. Preheat your oven to 350 °F
2. Bake almonds and cashews for 12 minutes
3. Let them cool
4. Transfer to a food processor and add remaining ingredients
5. Add oil and keep blending until smooth
6. Serve and enjoy!

NUTRITION: Calories: 205 Fat: 19g Carbohydrates: g Protein: 2.8g

231. Nut and Chia Mix

Preparation Time: 10 minutes

Cooking Time: 0 minute

Servings: 1

INGREDIENTS

- 1 tablespoon chia seeds
- 2 cups of water
- 1-ounce Macadamia nuts
- 1-2 packets Stevia, optional
- 1-ounce hazelnuts

DIRECTIONS

1. Add all the listed ingredients to a blender.
2. Blend on high until smooth and creamy.
3. Enjoy your smoothie.

NUTRITION: Calories: 452 Fat: 43g Carbohydrates: 15g Protein: 9g

232. Hearty Cucumber Bites

Preparation Time: 5 minutes

Cooking Time: 0 minute

Servings: 4

INGREDIENTS

- 1 (8 ounces) cream cheese container, low fat
- 1 tablespoon bell pepper, diced
- 1 tablespoon shallots, diced
- 1 tablespoon parsley, chopped
- 2 cucumbers
- Pepper to taste

DIRECTIONS

1. Take a bowl and add cream cheese, onion, pepper, parsley
2. Peel cucumbers and cut in half
3. Remove seeds and stuff with the cheese mix
4. Cut into bite-sized portions and enjoy!

NUTRITION: Calories: 85 Fat: 4g Carbohydrates: 2g Protein: 3g

233. Hearty Almond Bread

Preparation Time: 15 minutes

Cooking Time: 60 minutes

Servings: 8

INGREDIENTS

- 3 cups almond flour
- 1 teaspoon baking soda
- 2 teaspoons baking powder
- ¼ teaspoon sunflower seeds
- ¼ cup almond milk
- ½ cup + 2 tablespoons olive oil
- 3 whole eggs

DIRECTIONS

1. Preheat your oven to 300 ° F
2. Take a 9x5 inch loaf pan and grease, keep it on the side
3. Add the listed ingredients to a bowl and pour the batter into the loaf pan
4. Bake for 60 minutes
5. Once baked, remove this from oven and let it cool
6. Slice and serve!

NUTRITION: Calories: 277 Fat: 21g Carbohydrates: 7g Protein: 10g

234. Medjool Balls

Preparation Time: 5 minutes + 20 minutes chill time

Cooking Time: 2-3 minutes

Servings: 4

INGREDIENTS

- 3 cups Medjool dates, chopped
- 12 ounces brewed coffee
- 1 cup pecan, chopped
- ½ cup coconut, shredded
- ½ cup of cocoa powder

DIRECTIONS

1. Soak dates in warm coffee for 5 minutes
2. Remove dates from coffee and mash them, making a fine smooth mixture
3. Stir in the remaining ingredients (except cocoa powder) and form small balls out of the mixture
4. Coat with cocoa powder, serve and enjoy!

NUTRITION: Calories: 265 Fat: 12g Carbohydrates: 43g Protein 3g

235. Blueberry Pudding

Preparation Time: 20 minutes

Cooking Time: 0 minute

Servings: 4

INGREDIENTS

- 2 cups of frozen blueberries
- 2 teaspoon of lime zest, grated freshly
- 20 drops of liquid stevia
- ½ teaspoon of fresh ginger, grated freshly
- 4 tablespoon of fresh lime juice
- 10 tablespoons of water

DIRECTIONS

1. Add all of the listed ingredients to a blender (except blueberries) and pulse the mixture well
2. Transfer the mix into small serving bowls and chill the bowls
3. Serve with a topping of blueberries
4. Enjoy!

NUTRITION: Calories: 166 Fat: 13g Carbohydrates: 13g Protein: 1.7g

236. Chia Seed Pumpkin Pudding

Preparation Time: 10-15 minutes/ overnight chill time

Cooking Time: 0 minute

Servings: 4

INGREDIENTS

- 1 cup maple syrup
- 2 teaspoons pumpkin spice
- 1 cup pumpkin puree
- 1 ¼ cup of almond milk
- ½ cup chia seeds

DIRECTIONS

1. Add all of the ingredients to a bowl and gently stir
2. Let it refrigerate overnight or for at least 15 minutes
3. Top with your desired ingredients such as blueberries, almonds, etcetera.
4. Serve and enjoy!

NUTRITION: Calories: 230 Fat: 10g Carbohydrates:22g Protein:11g

237. Parsley Souffle

Preparation Time: 5 minutes

Cooking Time: 6 minutes

Servings: 5

INGREDIENTS

- 2 whole eggs
- 1 fresh red chili pepper, chopped
- 2 tablespoons coconut cream
- 1 tablespoon fresh parsley, chopped
- Sunflower seeds to taste

DIRECTIONS

1. Preheat your oven to 390 °F
2. Almond butter two soufflé dishes
3. Add the ingredients to a blender and mix well
4. Divide batter into soufflé dishes and bake for 6 minutes
5. Serve and enjoy!

NUTRITION: Calories: 108 Fat: 9g Carbohydrates: 9g Protein: 6g

238. Mug Cake Popper

Preparation Time: 5 minutes

Cooking Time: 5 minutes

Servings: 2

INGREDIENTS

- 2 tablespoons almond flour
- 1 tablespoon flaxseed meal
- 1 tablespoon almond butter
- 1 tablespoon cream cheese
- 1 large egg
- 1 bacon, cooked and sliced
- ½ jalapeno pepper
- ½ teaspoon baking powder
- ¼ teaspoon sunflower seeds

DIRECTIONS

1. Take a frying pan and place it over medium heat
2. Add sliced bacon and cook until they have a crispy texture
3. Take a microwave proof container and mix all of the listed ingredients (including cooked bacon), clean the sides
4. Microwave for 75 seconds making sure to put your microwave to high power
5. Take out the cup and slam it against a surface to take the cake out
6. Garnish with a bit of jalapeno and serve!

NUTRITION: Calories: 429 Fat: 38g Carbohydrates: 6g Protein: 16g

239. Cheesecake Bites

Preparation Time: 10 minutes

Cooking Time: 5 minutes

Servings: 16

INGREDIENTS

- 8-ounce cream cheese
- 1/2 teaspoon vanilla
- 1/4 cup swerve

DIRECTIONS

1. Add all ingredients into the mixing bowl and blend until well combined.
2. Place bowl into the fridge for 1 hour.
3. Remove bowl from the fridge. Make small balls from cheese mixture and place them on a baking dish.
4. Serve and enjoy.

NUTRITION: Calories 50 Fat 4.9 g Carbohydrates 0.4 g Sugar 0.1 g Protein 1.1 g Cholesterol 16 mg

240. Keto Mint Ginger Tea

Preparation Time: 5 minutes

Cooking Time: 5 minutes

Servings: 1

INGREDIENTS

- 1 1/2 tablespoon fresh mint leaves
- 1 cup of water
- 1/2 tablespoon fresh ginger, grated
- 1 teaspoon ground turmeric

DIRECTIONS

1. Add mint, ginger, and turmeric in boiling water.
2. Stir to turmeric dissolved.
3. Strain and serve.

NUTRITION: Calories 19 Fat 0.3 g Carbohydrates 4 g Sugar 0.3 g Protein 0.5 g Cholesterol 0 mg

241. Keto Brownie

Preparation Time: 10 minutes

Cooking Time: 20 minutes

Servings: 4

INGREDIENTS

- 2 tablespoon unsweetened cocoa powder
- 1/2 cup almond butter, melted
- 1 cup banana, overripe & mashed
- 1 scoop vanilla protein powder
- 1/2 teaspoon vanilla

DIRECTIONS

1. Preheat the oven to 350 F.
2. Line baking dish with parchment paper and set aside.
3. Add all ingredients into the blender and blend until smooth.
4. Pour in the batter into the prepared dish and then bake for 20 minutes.
5. Slice and serve.

NUTRITION: Calories 81 Fat 2 g Carbohydrates 10 g Sugar 5.2 g Protein 7 g Cholesterol 15 mg

242. Grilled Peach Sundaes

Preparation Time: 5 minutes

Cooking Time: 0 minute

Servings: 1

INGREDIENTS

- 1 tablespoon toasted unsweetened coconut
- 1 teaspoon canola oil
- 2 peaches, halved and pitted
- 2 scoops non-fat vanilla yogurt, frozen

DIRECTIONS

1. Brush the peaches with oil and grill until tender.
2. Place peach halves on a bowl and top with frozen yogurt and coconut.

NUTRITION: Calories: 61; carbs: 2g; protein: 2g; fats: 6g; phosphorus: 32mg; potassium: 85mg; sodium: 30mg

243. Belgian Waffle with Fruits

Preparation Time: 10 minutes

Cooking Time: 25 minutes

Servings: 6

INGREDIENTS

- Eggs – 2 larges
- Cake flour – 2 cups
- Baking soda – ¾ teaspoon
- Sour cream – ¾ cup
- 1% low-fat milk – ¾ cup
- Vanilla extract – 2 teaspoons
- Unsalted butter – 4 tablespoons
- Granulated sugar – 2 tablespoons
- Powdered sugar – 6 tablespoons

DIRECTIONS

1. Start by heating the waffle iron.
2. Now take a large mixing bowl and add in the baking soda and cake flour. Mix well and set aside.
3. Take 2 medium bowls and separate the egg whites and the yolks.
4. Add the vanilla extract and sour cream to the bowl with the egg yolks and whisk well. Add the melted butter and mix well.
5. Take the second bowl with the egg whites. Using a mixer on medium speed, beat the eggs to form soft peaks.
6. Add in the granulated sugar and beat for another 3-4 minutes to form stiff peaks.
7. Whisk together the flour mixture and sour cream mixture to combine well.
8. Add in the egg white mixture and gently fold through.
9. Add approximately ½ cup of batter to the heated waffle iron and close the iron.
10. Cook the mixture for 3 minutes. Once done, empty onto a serving platter.
11. Garnish with powdered sugar, fresh berries, syrup, and whipped cream.

NUTRITION: Carbohydrates – 50 g Protein – 8 g Fat – 15 g Sodium – 204 mg Cholesterol – 98 mg Potassium – 151 mg Calcium – 81 mg Phosphorus – 121 mg Fiber – 1 g

244. Spicy Broccoli macaroni

Preparation Time: 10 minutes

Cooking Time: 25 minutes

Servings: 2

INGREDIENTS

- 1 cup macaroni boiled
- 2 teaspoon garlic, chopped
- 1/2 teaspoon red chilies, chopped
- ¼ cup broccoli
- pepper
- olive oil

DIRECTIONS

1. Heat oil in a pan and sauté the garlic.
2. Add red chilies. Season with salt and pepper.
3. Add broccoli and cook for two minutes.
4. Add boiled macaroni.
5. Cook for 2-3 minutes. Serve hot.

NUTRITION: Calories 102, Total Fat 4.6g, Saturated Fat 1.1g, Cholesterol 3mg, Sodium 35mg, Total Carbohydrate 11.9g, Dietary Fiber 0.8g, Total Sugar 0.3g, Protein 3.4g, Calcium 39mg, Iron 0mg, Potassium 39mg, Phosphorus 10 mg

245. Quick Quiche

Preparation Time: 15 minutes

Cooking Time: 35 minutes

Servings: 2

INGREDIENTS

- 1 teaspoon olive oil
- 1 egg white, beaten
- 1 tablespoon finely chopped onion
- ¼ teaspoon black pepper
- ¼ cup all-purpose flour
- ½ cup soy milk

DIRECTIONS

1. Preheat oven to 350 degrees F. and then lightly grease a 9-inch pie pan.

2. Combine egg white, olive oil, onion, black pepper, flour and soy milk; whisk together until smooth; pour into pie pan.
3. Bake in preheated oven for 30-35 minutes, until set. Serve hot or cold.

NUTRITION: Calories 121, Total Fat 3.6g, Saturated Fat 0.5g, Cholesterol 0mg, Sodium 48mg, Total Carbohydrate 16.5g, Dietary Fiber 1g, Total Sugar 2.8g, Protein 5.5g, Calcium 21mg, Iron 1mg, Potassium 126mg, Phosphorus 90 mg

246. Chocolate Trifle

Preparation time: 20 minutes

Cooking time: 15 minutes

Servings: 4

INGREDIENTS:

- 1 small plain sponge swiss roll
- 3 oz. custard powder
- 5 oz. hot water
- 16 oz. canned mandarins
- 3 tablespoons sherry
- 5 oz. double cream
- 4 chocolate squares, grated

DIRECTION:

1. Whisk the custard powder with water in a bowl until dissolved.
2. In a bowl, mix the custard well until it becomes creamy and let it sit for 15 minutes.
3. Spread the swiss roll and cut it in 4 squares.
4. Place the swiss roll in the 4 serving cups.
5. Top the swiss roll with mandarin, custard, cream, and chocolate.
6. Serve.

NUTRITION: Calories 315 Total Fat 13.5g Cholesterol 43mg Sodium 185mg Protein 2.9g Calcium 61mg Phosphorous 184mg Potassium 129mg

247. Pineapple Meringues

Preparation time: 10 minutes

Cooking time: 0 minutes

Servings: 4

INGREDIENTS:

- 4 meringue nests
- 8 oz. crème fraiche
- 2 oz. stem ginger, chopped
- 8 oz. can pineapple chunks

DIRECTION:

1. Place the meringue nests on the serving plates.
2. Whisk the ginger with crème Fraiche and pineapple chunks.
3. Divide this the pineapple mixture over the meringue nests.
4. Serve.

NUTRITION: Calories 312 Cholesterol 0mg Sodium 41mg Protein 2.3g Calcium 3mg Phosphorous 104mg Potassium 110mg

248. Baked Custard

Preparation time: 15 minutes

Cooking time: 30 minutes

Servings: 1

INGREDIENTS:

- 1/2 cup milk
- 1 egg, beaten
- 1/8 teaspoon nutmeg
- 1/8 teaspoon vanilla
- Sweetener, to taste
- 1/2 cup water

DIRECTION:

1. Lightly warm up the milk in a pan, then whisk in the egg, nutmeg, vanilla and sweetener.
2. Pour this custard mixture into a ramekin.
3. Place the ramekin in a baking pan and pour ½ cup water into the pan.
4. Bake the custard for 30 minutes at 325 degrees F.
5. Serve fresh.

NUTRITION: Calories 127 Total Fat 7g Cholesterol 174mg Sodium 119mg Calcium 169mg Phosphorous 309mg Potassium 171mg

249. Strawberry Pie

Preparation time: 15 minutes

Cooking time: 25 minutes

Servings: 6

INGREDIENTS:

- 1 unbaked (9 inches) pie shell
- 4 cups strawberries, fresh
- 1 cup of brown Swerve
- 3 tablespoons arrowroot powder
- 2 tablespoons lemon juice
- 8 tablespoons whipped cream topping

DIRECTION:

1. Spread the pie shell in the pie pan and bake it until golden brown.
2. Now mash 2 cups of strawberries with the lemon juice, arrowroot powder, and Swerve in a bowl.

3. Add the mixture to a saucepan and cook on moderate heat until it thickens.
4. Allow the mixture to cool then spread it in the pie shell.
5. Slice the remaining strawberries and spread them over the pie filling.
6. Refrigerate for 1 hour then garnish with whipped cream.
7. Serve fresh and enjoy.

NUTRITION: Calories 236 Total Fat 11.1g Cholesterol 3mg Sodium 183mg Protein 2.2g Calcium 23mg Phosphorous 47.2mg Potassium 178mg

250. Easy Turnip Puree

Preparation Time: 10 minutes

Cooking Time: 12 minutes

Servings: 4

INGREDIENTS:

- 1 1/2 lbs. turnips, peeled and chopped
- 1 tsp dill
- 3 bacon slices, cooked and chopped
- 2 tbsp fresh chives, chopped

DIRECTIONS:

1. Add turnip into the boiling water and cook for 12 minutes. Drain well and place in a food processor.
2. Add dill and process until smooth.
3. Transfer turnip puree into the bowl and top with bacon and chives.
4. Serve and enjoy.

NUTRITION: Calories 127 Fat 6 g Carbohydrates 11.6 g Sugar 7 g Protein 6.8 g Cholesterol 16 mg

251. Spinach Bacon Bake

Preparation Time: 10 minutes

Cooking Time: 45 minutes

Servings: 6

INGREDIENTS:

- 10 eggs
- 3 cups baby spinach, chopped
- 1 tbsp olive oil
- 8 bacon slices, cooked and chopped
- 2 tomatoes, sliced
- 2 tbsp chives, chopped
- Pepper
- Salt

DIRECTIONS:

1. Preheat the oven to 350 F.
2. Spray a baking dish with cooking spray and set aside.
3. Heat oil in a pan.
4. Add spinach and cook until spinach wilted.
5. In a mixing bowl, whisk eggs and salt. Add spinach and chives and stir well.
6. Pour egg mixture into the baking dish.
7. Top with tomatoes and bacon and bake for 45 minutes.
8. Serve and enjoy.

NUTRITION: Calories 273 Fat 20.4 g Carbohydrates 3.1 g Sugar 1.7 g Protein 19.4 g Cholesterol 301 mg

252. Healthy Spinach Tomato Muffins

Preparation Time: 10 minutes

Cooking Time: 20 minutes

Servings: 12

INGREDIENTS:

- 12 eggs
- 1/2 tsp Italian seasoning
- 1 cup tomatoes, chopped
- 4 tbsp water
- 1 cup fresh spinach, chopped
- Pepper
- Salt

DIRECTIONS:

1. Preheat the oven to 350 F.
2. Spray a muffin tray with cooking spray and set aside.
3. In a mixing bowl, whisk eggs with water, Italian seasoning, pepper, and salt.
4. Add spinach and tomatoes and stir well.
5. Pour egg mixture into the prepared muffin tray and bake for 20 minutes.
6. Serve and enjoy.

NUTRITION: Calories 67 Fat 4.5 g Carbohydrates 1 g Sugar 0.8 g Protein 5.7 g Cholesterol 164 mg

CONCLUSION

The proper renal diet can really help kidneys functioning longer, and it has only more restrictions on proteins and table salt, while restrictions to phosphorous and potassium can be needed if the levels of blood rise and the signs of accumulation become too evident.

Each recipe listed will help you achieve your health and fitness goals and provide most of the nutrients that the body needs to function. Your body won't be deprived of any micronutrient or macronutrient. The Low sodium will also assist in striking the right balance between saturated and unsaturated fats.

Don'ts of a kidney diet

- Don't utilize nourishment plans which have generous amounts of mineral salts particularly oxalate salts from calcium, phosphorus, manganese. These mineral components can cause quicker kidney degeneration and extreme weakness in kidney working.
- Don't eat overabundance segments of nourishments that have high convergences of immersed fats, burgers, and red meat or any handled food sources.
- Don't drink liquor, caffeinated beverages, or refreshments with high sugar content-both may exhaust the liver and intensify or cause degeneration of the kidney issue.
- Don't devour sugary substances, for example, tidbits, deserts, or confections since they cause a lack of hydration and exhaust the kidney simply like salts.
- Do not take a wide range of common red meat in your kidney diet-hamburger, pork, bacon, or lamb and their options seared, restored, or prepared meats, rather search for lean white meat from poultry.
- Do not utilize any fake sugars while planning nourishments since they have no healthful advantages
- Do not utilize margarine or mayonnaise yet options, for example, an avocado natural product on the off chance that you need to devour fat.
- Do not eat a bigger number of helpings than should be expected particularly to delights, for example, fries, frozen yogurts, soft drinks, and other sweet nourishments and a wide range of handled or canned nourishments
- Don't devour a greater number of starches than should be expected in your kidney diet and this incorporates such carbs like pasta, white rice, scones, white sugar, white rice, and pasta.
- Do's of a kidney diet
- Do take enough liquids to keep centralization of minerals, for example, calcium and sodium on the kidney low. These will to guarantee appropriate kidney working, counteract lack of hydration which is the regular reason for kidney stones in the renal cylinders, and detoxify the kidney also.
- Do embrace a reasonable eating regimen for a renal illness which contains crisp vegetables, entire grains, and lean meat just as water. Greens and natural products plentiful in nutrients improve cell digestion and the working of organs.
- Do take fiber or fuse fiber-rich suppers and entire grains in your renal eating routine which are low in carbs however advance general wellbeing and lift kidney working.
- Do eat modestly and create smart dieting propensities to guarantee that your body gets the correct stock of minerals and supplements.
- Do eat vegetables and organic products as regularly as you can and consolidate them in your kidney diet intend to help your invulnerability and cell digestion
- Do utilize low-fat milk items, for example, milk powder on the off chance that you need to utilize them as opposed to utilizing milk with cream or fat.
- Do utilize monounsaturated fat or normal fat when cooking and lower the measure of fat that you expend every day in your dinners.

- Do grasp dynamic and energetic life to decrease heftiness or strange weight, help working of renal eating routine, and advance great body digestion and kidney working. Exercise guarantees blood dissemination to kidney and lifts exercises, for example, detoxification and separating.
- Carbohydrates are important for energy and need to be taken in the right quantities. However, you should avoid refined ones. You should try to use as many whole grains and unrefined forms of carbohydrates as possible.
- Table salt should be used only for cooking and remember that excessive salt causes retention and stress to the kidneys. Salty foods should be avoided as well: no sausages, no snacks, no tinned food.
- There is also the level of phosphorus which needs to be monitored carefully, avoiding colored drinks like colas and food with a high level of potassium such as bananas, citrus fruits, apricots, dark leafy green vegetables should be avoided too, especially if blood levels rise.
- Take into consideration also Omega 3 fats which are important in your diet but avoid trans-fats and hydrolyzed fats.
- Low sodium meals cooked in slow cookers won't just save your precious time but will also reduce the hassle of being physically present in the kitchen. You come home from work or play to delicious and healthy meals. It is recommended to do the preparation for cooking in advance, preferably the previous night. Next morning all you have to do is dump the meals in a slow cooker, adjust the heat settings and that is it!

Made in United States
North Haven, CT
09 October 2023

42547758R00052